Chest X-Ray in Clinical Practice

Rita Joarder · Neil Crundwell
Editors

Chest X-Ray in Clinical Practice

Springer

Editors
Dr. Rita Joarder
Conquest Hospital
The Ridge
St. Leonards-On-Sea
East Sussex
United Kingdom TN37 7RD
Rita.Joarder@esht.nhs.uk

Dr. Neil Crundwell
Conquest Hospital
The Ridge
St. Leonards-On-Sea
East Sussex
United Kingdom TN37 7RD
Neil.Crundwell@esht.nhs.uk

ISBN 978-1-84882-098-2 e-ISBN 978-1-84882-099-9
DOI 10.1007/978-1-84882-099-9
Springer Dordrecht Heidelberg London New York

British Library Cataloguing in Publication Data
A catalogue record for this book is available from the British Library

Library of Congress Control Number: 2009926729

Cover design: eStudio Calamar S.L.

Printed on acid-free paper

Springer is part of Springer Science+Business Media (www.springer.com)

'To Martin, Alfred, Arnold, and Freddie, for your unceasing support and inspiration' Rita Joarder

'To Lesley and Sebastian for showing me life's beautiful things' Neil Crundwell

Preface

The chest radiograph (chest X-ray) is the most commonly requested examination, and it is probably the hardest plain film to interpret correctly. Accurate interpretation can greatly influence patient management in the acute setting. It is, however, often performed out of hours and the interpretation is undertaken by relatively junior members of staff with no immediate senior support or radiological input. Despite the increasing availability of more complex radiological investigations, the chest X-ray continues to be requested as a first-line investigation and this is likely to continue.

The structure of this book derives from many teaching sessions that have been given to junior doctors and medical students. The authors have found that, in general, teaching regarding chest X-ray interpretation had lacked a formal structured approach, and junior doctors and medical students found interpreting a chest X-ray difficult. Giving them a structured approach allowed them to feel they could tackle interpretation with more confidence.

We aim to provide a portable handbook for junior doctors. The structure is based upon those lectures that the authors have given. The book itself is intended to be easily accessible and to help this we have included tables containing the key teaching points, to allow easy reference. We have included extensive examples of common pathologies. This book is, however, not an exhaustive work of reference.

We have included basic information on how a chest X-ray is performed and how such performance factors can affect the quality of the image. We consider the implications of radiation dose and give details of basic normal anatomy. We then explain why normal structures appear as they do on the chest

X-ray. The ability to interpret the normal is key to interpreting the abnormal and we explain why abnormalities create the imaging features they do.

Using a structured logical approach, we focus on both anatomical abnormality and more generalized patterns of lung disease.

Our ultimate aim is to equip the reader with a confident, simple but logical approach to chest X-ray interpretation.

R. Joarder
N. Crundwell

Acknowledgments

We would like to acknowledge Christina Worley for all her hard work in preparing the manuscript.

We would also like to acknowledge the following for their valuable contribution to this book: Steve Page, DCR, MSc, Conquest Hospital, St Leonards-On-Sea, East Sussex, UK, and Andrew Develing, DipMDI, Conquest Hospital, St Leonards-On-Sea, East Sussex, UK

Contents

Part I

Chapter 1
Chest Radiography

It is important to understand how an X-ray image is generated. Artifacts and other pseudo-abnormalities can be much more easily explained if you are aware of how they may be created.

X-rays are high-frequency short wavelength electromagnetic radiation, which penetrate different tissues to differing extents. The X-ray beam, although very narrow, is divergent and does fan out, resulting in a slightly different amount of exposure in the center as opposed to the margins of the film.

Image generation is similar in principle to photography, with X-rays replacing light as the medium that "exposes" the film. In an X-ray image, areas of the film exposed to the beam appear dark/black. Areas of the film not exposed due to absorption of the beam by soft tissues appear white.

The relative position of the patient with regard to the X-ray beam and the film plays a fundamental role in the resulting image. A brief outline of the principles of radiographic positioning is now given.

The general principle for any radiographic examination is to position the body part under investigation as close to the imaging medium as possible. This is to avoid undue elongation or foreshortening of the body part. For the chest radiograph the same is true, and this examination can be carried out to demonstrate the lungs, ribs, mediastinum, and heart.

The basic projections and techniques can be modified to demonstrate each region of interest.

R. Joarder, N. Crundwell (eds.), *Chest X-Ray in Clinical Practice*,
DOI 10.1007/978-1-84882-099-9_1,

The main chest projections are the following:

1) Postero-anterior (PA) – the ray enters the posterior aspect of the patient and exits the anterior
2) Antero-posterior (AP) – the ray enters the anterior aspect and exits the posterior
3) Lateral
4) Obliques – either anterior or posterior – to demonstrate mediastinum or ribs
5) Penetrated postero-anterior
6) Inspiration/expiration postero-anterior – for pneumothorax, inhaled foreign bodies, or for diaphragmatic movement
7) Apical lordotic

1.1 Radiographic Technique

1.1.1 Postero-anterior (PA)

For the best results the patient should be erect (standing or seated) so the diaphragm is at its lowest position and engorgement of the pulmonary vessels is avoided.

Position the patient with the anterior surface of the chest against the upright film holder, with their median sagittal plane at right angles to the film. The top of the film should be positioned 5–8 cm above the patient's shoulders so that on full inspiration the entire apices are included. The patient's weight should be evenly distributed on the feet, and the patient's shoulders should not be raised or the apices will be obscured by clavicles (Fig. 1.1).

The patient's hands are placed with the posterior aspects on the back of the hips and elbows gently rolled forward until the shoulders are touching the film. This removes the scapulae from the lung fields. The film size must ensure the lateral edges of both lungs are included on the film and that on full inspiration both diaphragms are included on the inferior aspect of the film.

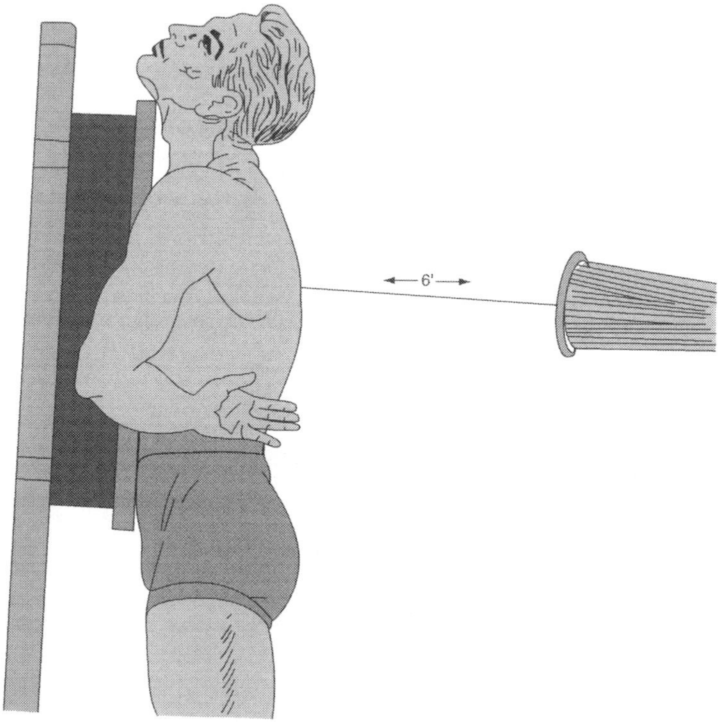

Figure 1.1. Patient position for PA CXR.

The central ray is projected at right angles to the film and centered at the level of the fourth thoracic vertebra, in the midline. The divergent rays allow for clearance of the dome of the diaphragm. The film is taken on full arrested inspiration, to demonstrate the greatest possible area of lung structure (Fig. 1.2).

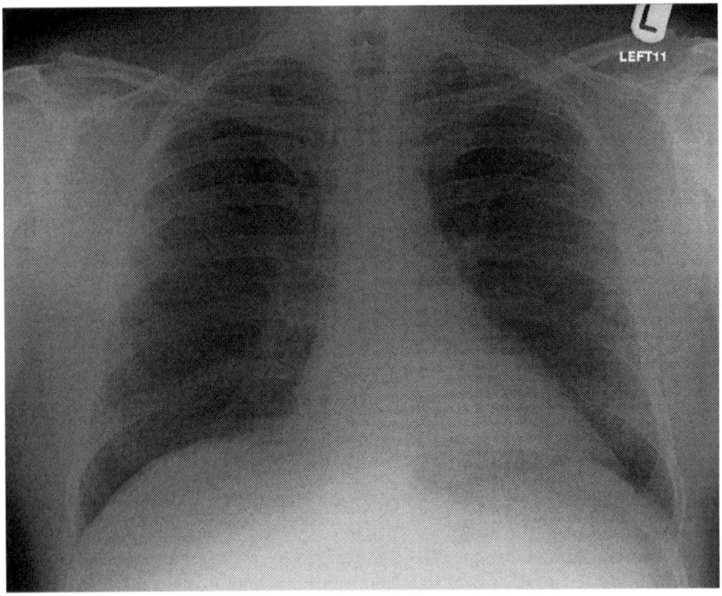

FIGURE 1.2. PA CXR.

1.1.1.1 Image Evaluation

1) The medial ends of the clavicles should be equidistant from the vertebral column
2) The trachea should be in the midline
3) The scapulae should be off the lung fields
4) There should be 10 posterior ribs visible above the diaphragm
5) Five centimeter of lung apices should be above the clavicles
6) Both costophrenic angles should be included on the film

1.1.2 Antero-posterior

The patient is positioned with their posterior aspect against the imaging plate, with the median sagittal plane at right angles to the film. The film is positioned 5–8 cm above the shoulder to allow apices to be included on the film, on full inspiration.

The backs of the patient's hands are placed on the backs of the hips and the shoulders rotated gently forward to remove scapulae from the film.

The central ray is projected at right angles to the film, in the midline of the patient, at the level of the sternal notch and the film exposed on arrested full inspiration.

1.1.3 Lateral

The patient is positioned with their side against the film – for cardiac examinations a left lateral (left side closest to the film) and for lung pathology the side under examination should be closest to the film (Fig. 1.3).

The median sagittal plane of the patient should be parallel to the film (to ensure the scapulae are superimposed) and the patient should stand with their feet slightly apart to maintain balance. The arms of the patient should be folded across their head, to clear the lungs.

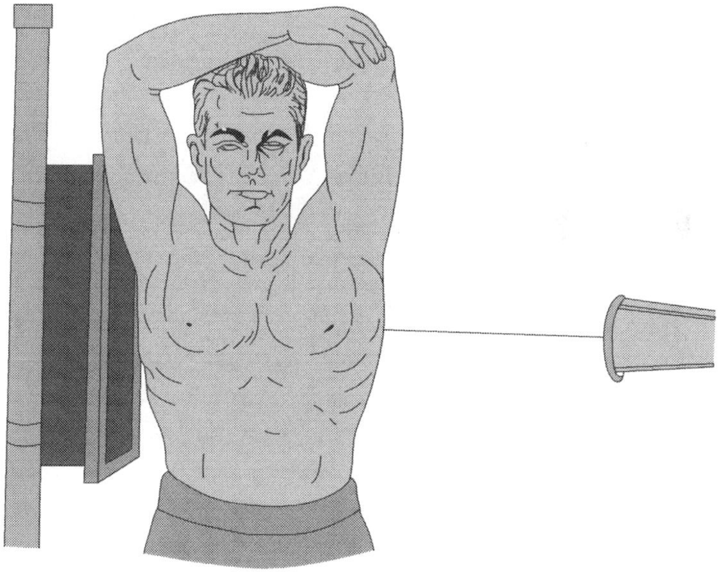

FIGURE 1.3. Patient position for lateral CXR.

The central ray is projected at right angles to the film and should be centered midway between the anterior and posterior skin surfaces, at the level of the fourth thoracic vertebra. The film should be taken on full arrested inspiration (Fig. 1.4).

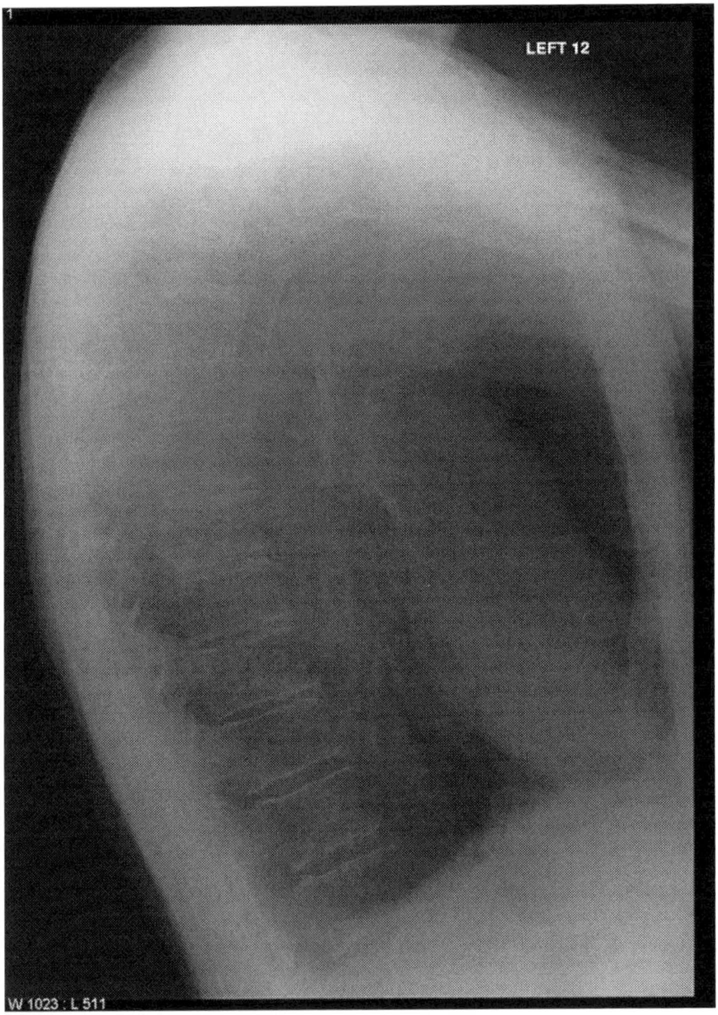

FIGURE 1.4. Lateral CXR.

1.1.3.1 Image Evaluation

1) The long axis of the body should be vertical.
2) There should not be any arms overlapping the lungs.
3) The posterior ribs should be superimposed.

1.1.4 Obliques

These are generally now only taken to demonstrate that the ribs and oblique views of the mediastinum are on the whole redundant.

i) Ribs 1–10

These projections can be taken in an antero-posterior or postero-anterior position depending on the site of the injury.

From the AP position the patient is rotated 45° with the affected side closest to the film and in contact with the film. The arm should be raised slightly away from the body and if possible placed behind the head.

The central ray should be at right angles to the film and be centered at the level of the sternal angle.

The film is taken on full arrested inspiration.

ii) Ribs 9–12

For the lowest four pairs of ribs it is most satisfactory to project them below the diaphragm. An antero-posterior projection taken to include the eighth thoracic vertebra to the third lumbar vertebra, on full arrested expiration, is the most efficient method.

The centering point is the level of the lower costal margin, in the midline (Fig. 1.5).

Antero-posterior or postero-anterior obliques where the patient is obliqued 45° to either side, depending on the site of the injury, can be carried out. This projects the injured rib as parallel to the film as possible. The film is again centered on the lower costal margin and taken on arrested expiration (Fig. 1.6).

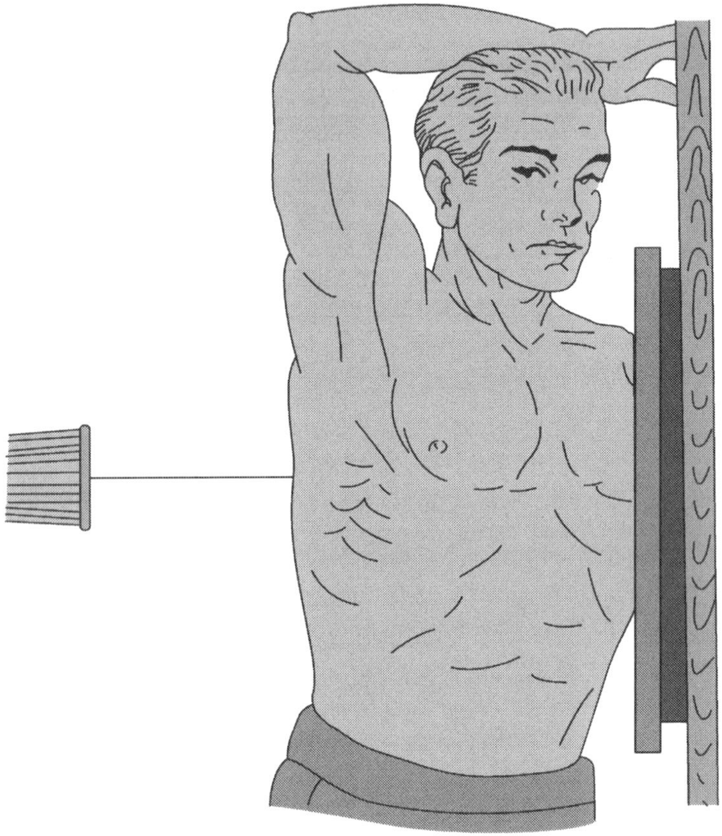

FIGURE 1.5. Patient position for left anterior oblique CXR.

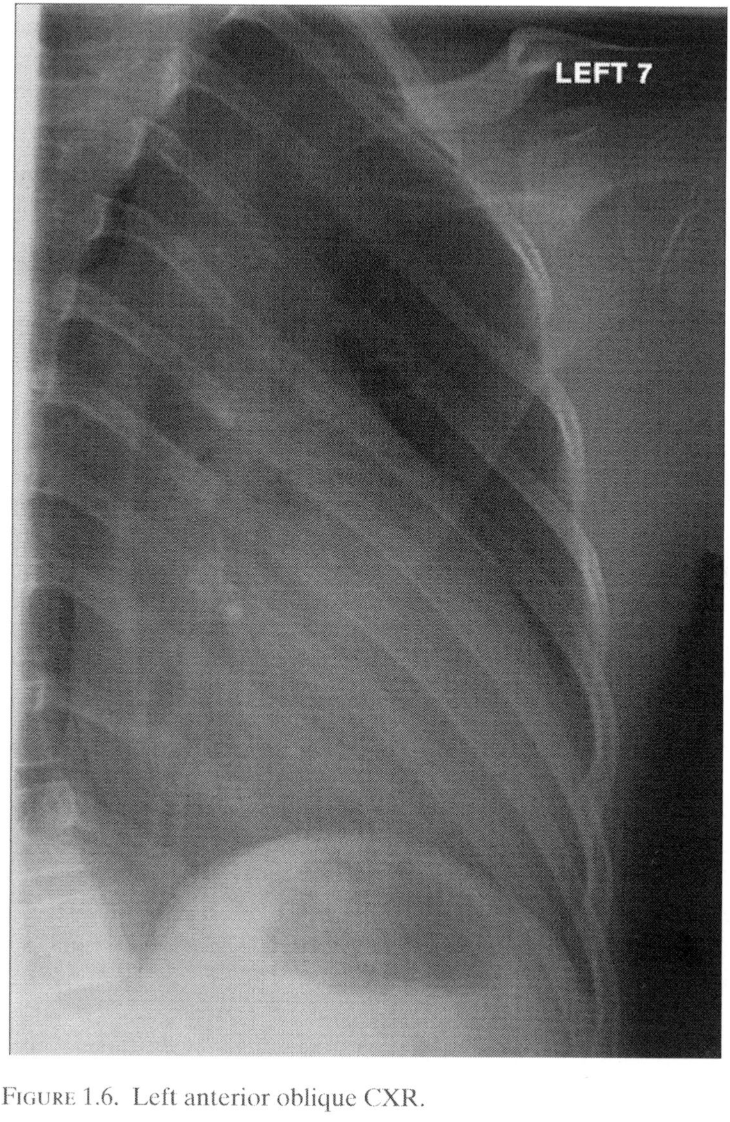

FIGURE 1.6. Left anterior oblique CXR.

1.1.5 Penetrated Postero-anterior

The patient is positioned as for the PA and the radiographic technique only varies in exposure factors. The additional penetration is used to demonstrate pathology behind the heart and should clearly demonstrate eight thoracic vertebrae.

1.1.6 Inspiration/Expiration Postero-anterior

The patient is positioned as for routine PA and radiographic technique only varies in phase of respiration.

Inspiration/expiration projections are used to demonstrate diaphragmatic travel, for inhaled foreign bodies, for pneumothorax, or for collapse of individual lobes.

1.1.7 Apical Lordotic

This projection is used to demonstrate the lung apices free from superimposition of the clavicles.

The patient stands with their median sagittal plane at right angles to the film, with their back against the film. They step forward 20–30 cm and lean back so that their shoulders are against the film.

The central ray is projected at right angles to the film, centered at the level of the sternal notch. The film is taken on full arrested inspiration.

1.1.7.1 Image Evaluation

1) The clavicles should lie above the apices.
2) The medial ends of the clavicles should be equidistant from the vertebral column.
3) The clavicles should be superimposing only the first rib.

1.2 Key Points

1) Proper radiographic technique is essential for the generation of diagnostically adequate chest X-rays.
2) Correct patient position is a key part of radiographic technique.
3) An understanding of image generation allows identification of artifacts and pseudo-abnormalities.

Chapter 2
The Normal Chest X-ray: An Approach to Interpretation

Being able to recognize normal appearances and structures as seen on a chest X-ray (CXR) is key to being able to correctly interpret any abnormal findings. In order to do this, we must first understand why we are able to see structures such as the heart border and the ribs as separate entities to surrounding tissues.

Different materials absorb X-rays to differing extents. Air absorbs very little of the X-ray beam. Structures such as the lungs, which are mostly air, will therefore allow a large amount of the X-ray beam to pass through, causing blackening of the film and therefore they appear as dark areas. Materials such as bone absorb much of the X-ray beam and there will be little blackening of the film. Consequently these areas will appear white. The more X-rays the material stops, the whiter its appearance on a plain film. All tissues stop X-rays to a greater or lesser extent with air and bone being at the extremes.

The difference in the amount of the X-ray beam that different tissues absorb is termed the attenuation. This difference in attenuation is what enables us to make out different structures on an X-ray film. For example, we see the border of the heart because it is adjacent to air-filled lung, the so-called silhouette sign. The attenuation of the heart is different from that of the air-filled lung and so the heart appears more opaque than the lung and a border is seen.

If material of a similar density to the heart, for example, a lung tumour or lymph nodes, forms adjacent to the heart, this

R. Joarder, N. Crundwell (eds.), *Chest X-Ray in Clinical Practice*,
DOI 10.1007/978-1-84882-099-9_2,

interface is lost and the border of the heart or mediastinal structure is lost. Structures that are not normally seen may become apparent by the interposition of air. For example, in a pneumothorax, air creates a new air/soft tissue interface and the pleural margin of the lung is seen.

The basic principle is that the difference in the amount of X-rays that different tissues absorb alters how white or dark they appear on the radiographic image. Adjacent structures which absorb X-rays to a different extent will therefore be of different density and this interface allows us to visualise structures (Fig. 2.1)

Before we start interpreting the chest X-ray, there are a few fundamental checks that need to be made. Always ensure that the X-ray has the correct patient name, unit number, and

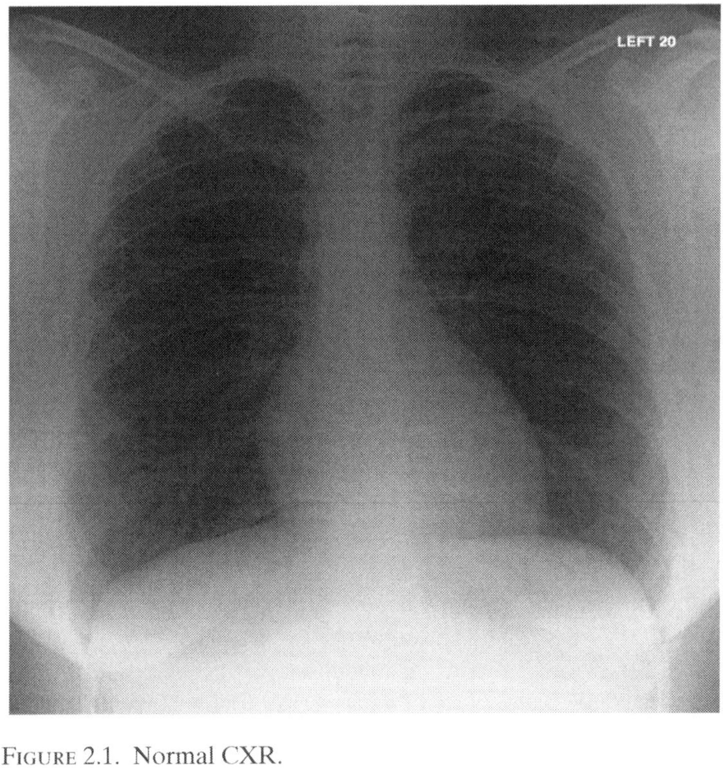

FIGURE 2.1. Normal CXR.

date of birth, and always ensure you check the date of the film that you are looking at. Most hospitals will now have a PACS (picture archiving and communication system) imaging system, but even so images can be inverted and the side marker should always be checked. If there is any doubt regarding the technical features of the film these should be checked with the radiographer.

It is important to ensure that the patient has been well positioned with respect to the film. Rotation of the patient will alter the appearance of the mediastinal structures and can make one lung look darker than the other. The positioning of the patient can be easily checked using the alignment of the medial ends of the clavicles with the posterior spinous processes. The spinous processes should be at equal distance from each clavicle.

In the ideal circumstance, chest X-rays are obtained in a PA (posterior anterior) projection. As described in Chapter 1, in order to do this the patient must be able to stand upright. In the acute setting this is often not possible, and many films are obtained in an AP (anterior posterior) position. This should be marked on the film. The apparent cardiothoracic ratio may be falsely elevated on an AP projection and care should be taken when interpreting the cardiac size.

Chest X-rays should be taken with a good inspiration, resulting in at least six ribs being visible anteriorly. An underexpanded chest can create the impression of lung abnormality, for example, mimicking pulmonary oedema.

2.1 Understanding Normal Anatomy

In order to be able to successfully interpret abnormalities on a chest X-ray, it is important to be able to interpret the normal anatomy. Remember that margins are seen on a radiograph due to a difference in the relative attenuation of adjacent structures.

Starting at the top of the left side of the mediastinum (Fig. 2.2), we see the aortic knuckle followed by the left pulmonary artery and the aortopulmonary window. This is the

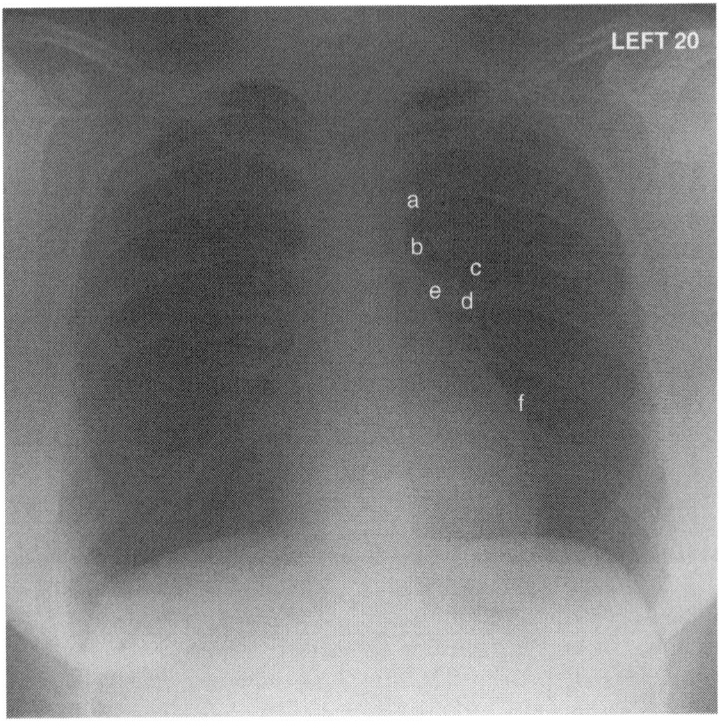

FIGURE 2.2. Normal CXR with left side annotated. (a) Aortic knuckle, (b) Aorto pulmonary window, (c) Left pulmonary artery, (d) Hilar point, (e) Left atrium, (f) Left ventricle.

space between the aorta and the pulmonary artery. Moving more inferiorly we see the hilar point. This is a radiological feature created by the overlap of the draining upper lobe pulmonary veins and the lower lobe pulmonary artery. Beneath this we see the left atrium and the left ventricle. Remember that we see these structures because the tissue adjacent to them is of lower radiographic density. So if we fail to see a clear hilar point, this suggests that there is a soft tissue abnormality in the region of the hilum.

If the patient is adequately positioned, the majority of the right heart border is made up of the right atrium, the right

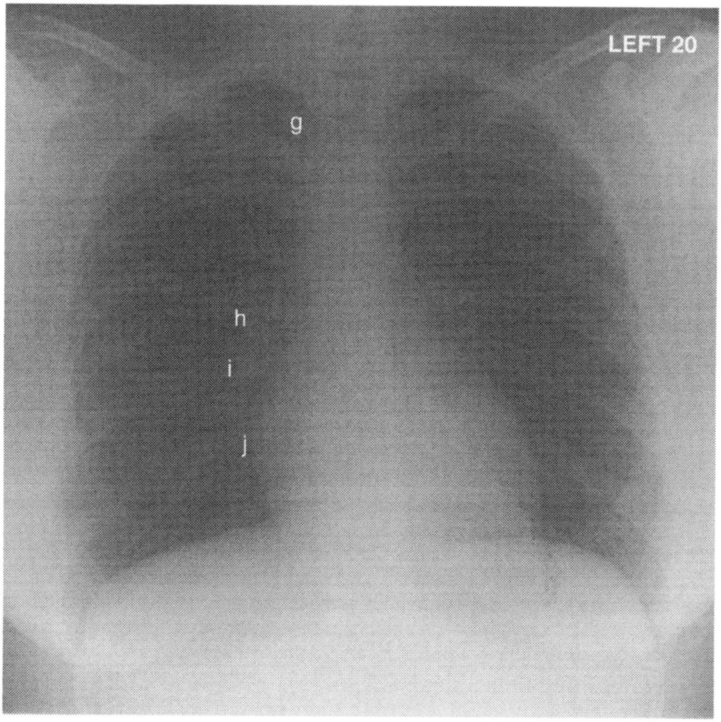

FIGURE 2.3. Normal CXR with right side annotated. (g) Right para tracheal region, (h) hilar point, (i) lower lobe pulmonary artery, (j) right atrium.

ventricle being a more anteriorly placed structure (Fig. 2.3). Being of similar density to the atrium, it cannot be separated.

As we pass more superiorly, we sometimes see the lateral margin of the superior vena cava in the right paratracheal region, particularly if the film is a little rotated. We then pass superiorly toward the apices, following the mediastinal contour and trachea, toward the cervical region.

In the normal chest X-ray, the lungs are predominantly black and a branching pattern of vessels is seen. Remember that there are three lobes in the right lung and two in the left (Figs. 2.4 a, b and c). There are fissures that separate these lobes and these may be visible as linear structures on the normal chest X-ray.

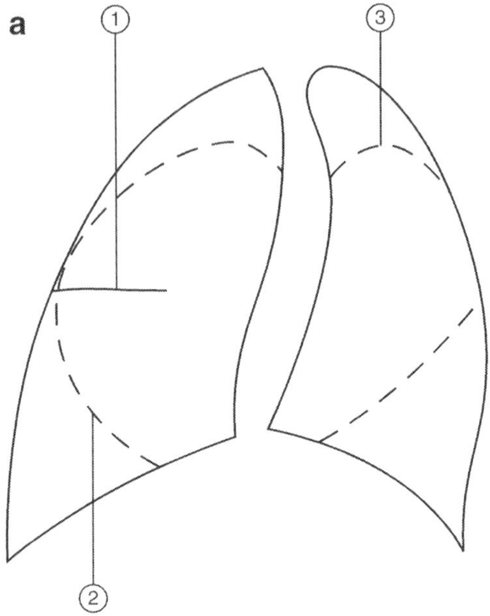

FIGURE 2.4. Diagram of lungs showing lobes. The right lung has three lobes, upper, middle and lower. These are separated by the oblique and horizontal fissures. The left lung has two lobes, upper and lower separated by the oblique fissure. Figure 2.4a (1) Horizontal fissure (2) Right oblique fissure, (3) Left oblique fissure. Figure 2.4b (1) Horizontal fissure (2) Right oblique fissure (3) Right upper lobe (4) Right middle lobe (5) Right lower lobe. Figure 2.4c (1) Left oblique fissure (2) Left upper lobe (3) Left lower lobe.

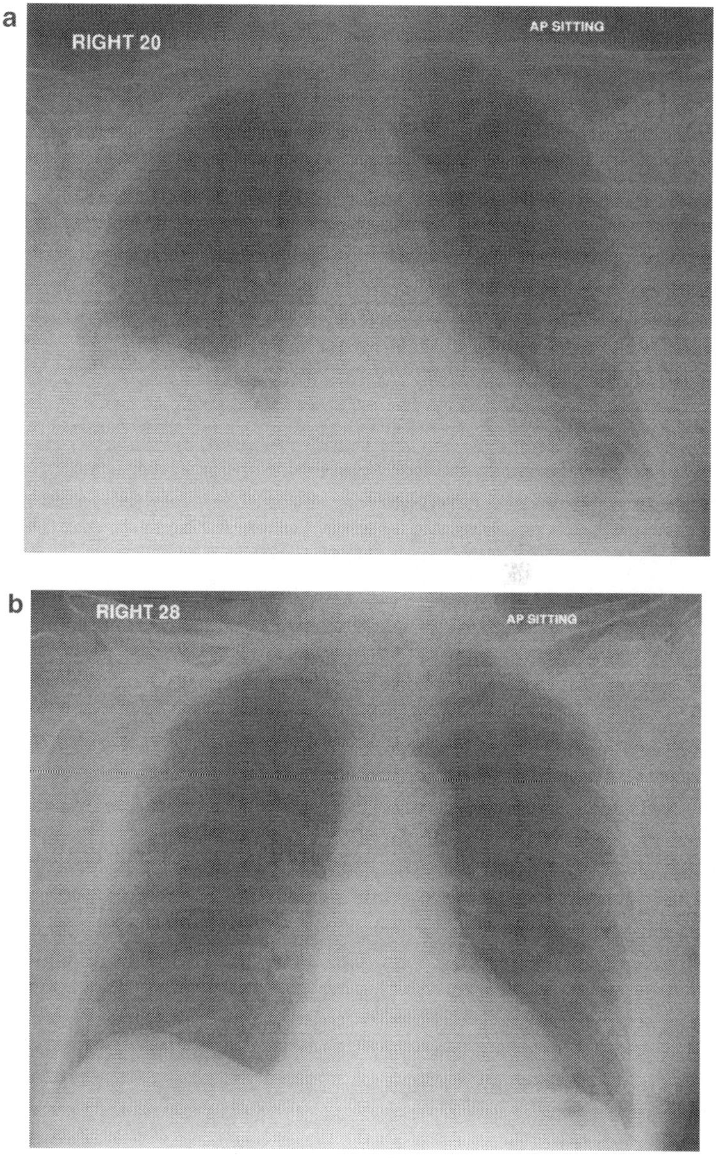

FIGURE 2.7. (a) Poor and (b) Good inspiration.

a

b

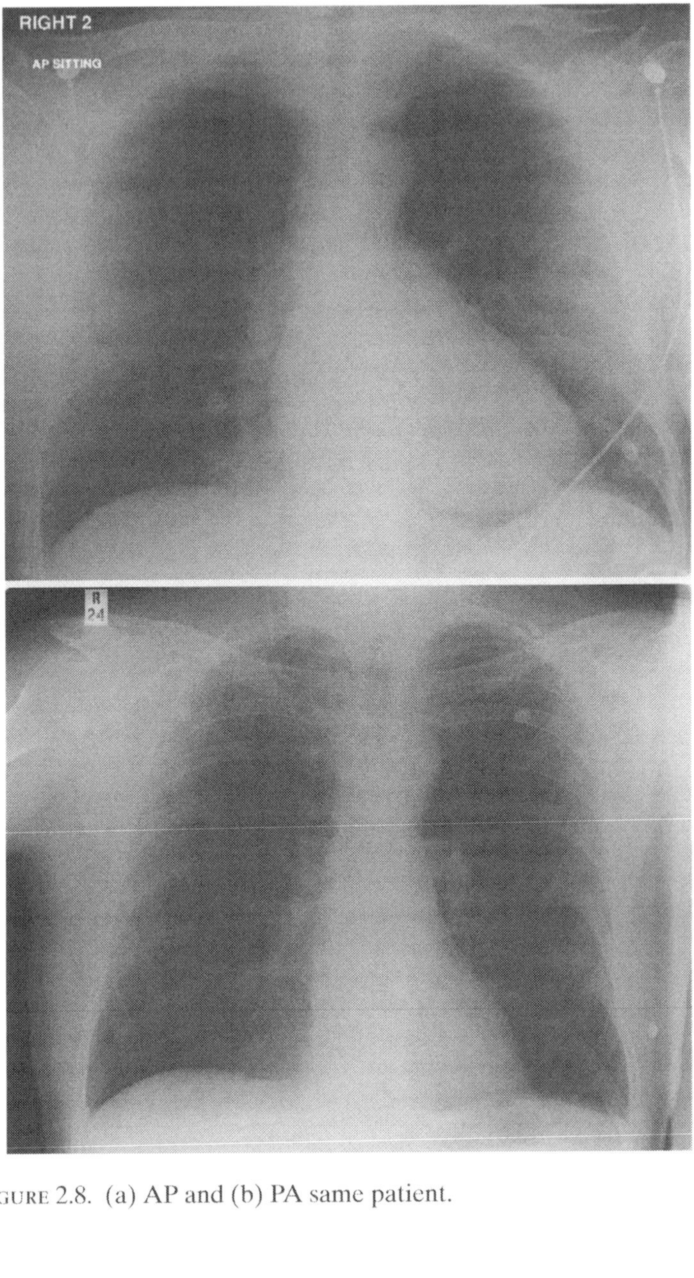

FIGURE 2.8. (a) AP and (b) PA same patient.

2.4 Key Points

1) The differing X-ray attenuation of different materials creates borders (silhouette sign).
2) Loss of normal anatomy suggests pathology.
3) Always check review areas.
4) Do not overinterpret pseudo-abnormalities.

Part II

Chapter 3
The Mediastinum and Hilar Regions

The mediastinum is divided into anterior, middle, and posterior regions, subdivided into superior and inferior regions (Fig. 3.1). We see the outline of the mediastinum because structures are adjacent to other structures of differing radiodensity. This is generally soft tissue against air.

While the hilar are not strictly part of the mediastinum they are intimately related to it and will be covered in this chapter.

When assessing the mediastinum, remember what the normal contour should look like and assess whether this can be seen. For example, if the posterior and anterior structures are still well defined, the lesion must be in the middle. Similarly if the middle and posterior structures are well defined, the lesion must lie in the anterior mediastinum, and so on. By using this principle, it can be established whether abnormalities are within the anterior, middle, or posterior regions.

Examples of common abnormalities are given to demonstrate the principles of interpretation of the mediastinum (Table 3.1).

R. Joarder, N. Crundwell (eds.), *Chest X-Ray in Clinical Practice*,
DOI 10.1007/978-1-84882-099-9_3,

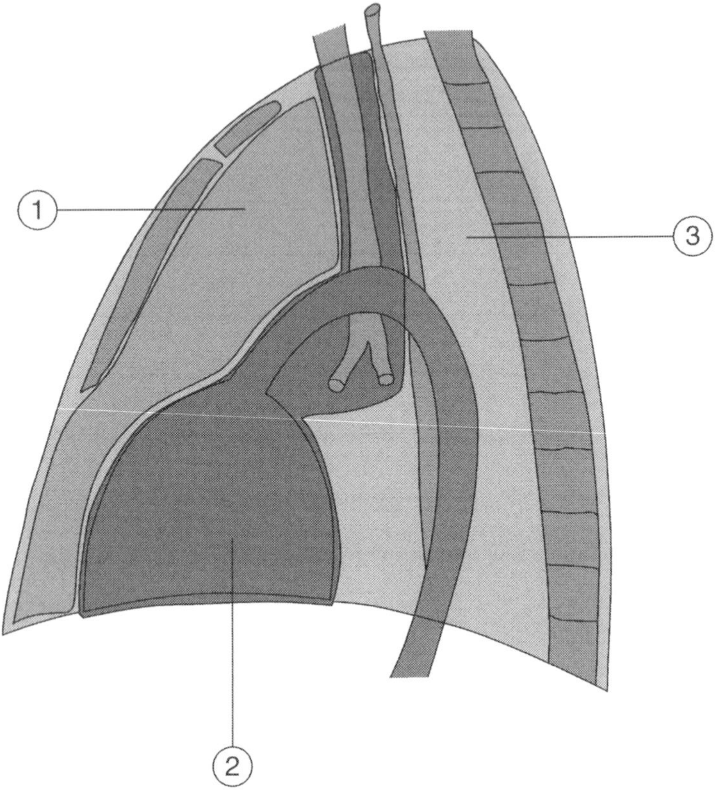

FIGURE 3.1. Diagram to show the anterior, middle, and posterior compartments of the mediastinum. (1) Anterior mediastinum; (2) middle mediastinum; (3) posterior mediastinum.

TABLE 3.1. Mediastinal masses.

Region	Pathology
Anterior mediastinum	Teratodermoid
	Thymoma
	Thyroid mass
	Lymphoma
Middle mediastinum	Lymphadenopathy
	Cardiac abnormality; atrial or ventricular enlargement, dextrocardia
	Pericardial abnormality; effusion, cyst
	Vascular abnormality; arch aortic aneurysm, aortic dissection
	Vascular variant; right-sided aortic arch, double aortic arch, left-sided SVC
	Tracheal abnormality; tumour, cyst
	Foregut duplication cyst; bronchogenic, oesophageal
Posterior mediastinum	Oesophageal abnormality; achalasia, neoplasia, hiatus hernia
	Vascular abnormality; descending aortic aneurysm
	Neurogenic neoplasm
	Paraspinal mass; abscess, metastasis
	Extramedullary hemopoiesis
	Foregut duplication cyst; neurenteric

3.1 Middle Mediastinum and Hilar Regions

The structures within the middle mediastinum include the heart and the hilar regions.

3.1.1 Cardiac Abnormality

3.1.1.1 Left Atrial Enlargement

The signs of left atrial enlargement include bulging of the left atrial appendage, an apparent double right heart border (Fig. 3.2a) and splaying of the carina (Fig. 3.2b). The normal

a

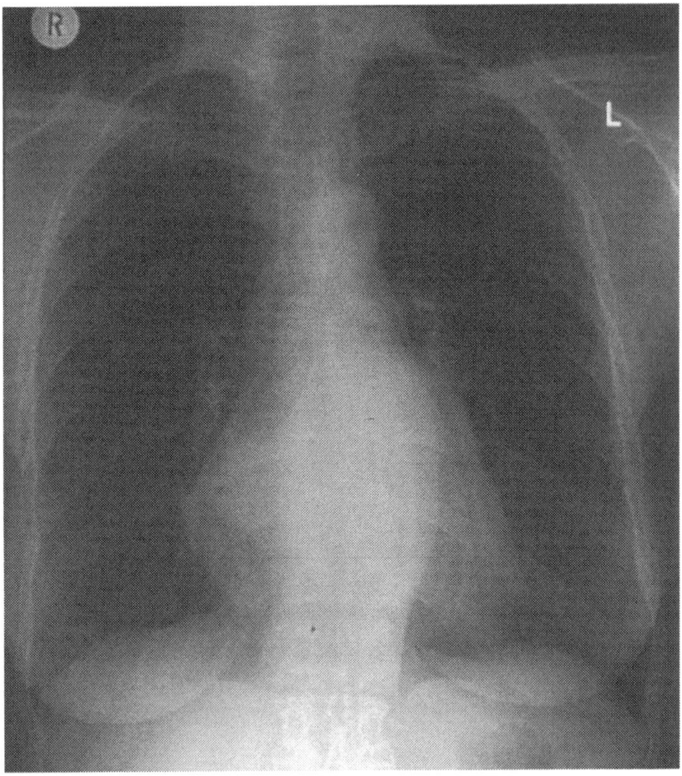

FIGURE 3.2a. Enlarged left atrium showing bulging left atrium and double right heart border.

b

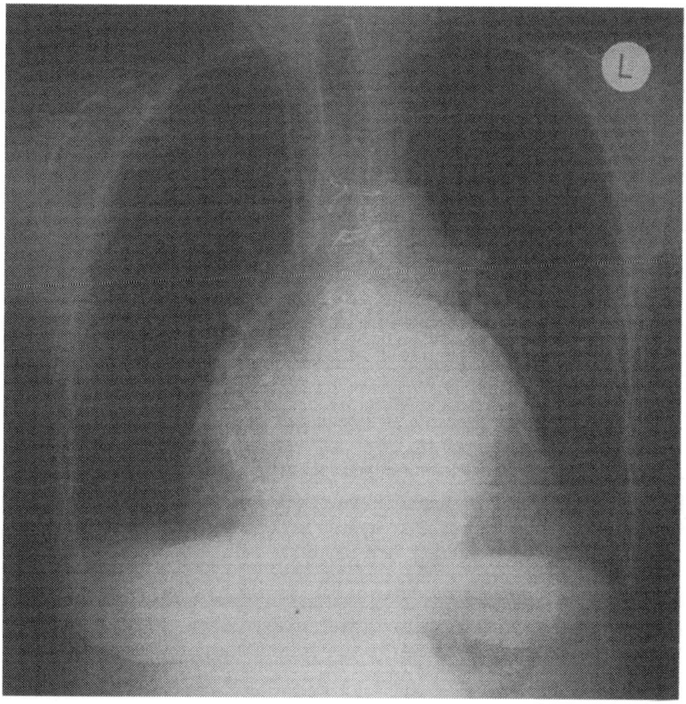

FIGURE 3.2b. Enlarged left atrium with bulging left atrium and splaying of the carina.

carinal angle is on average 70°. Patients may also have undergone treatment for the causes of left atrial enlargement, such as mitral valve replacement for mitral regurgitation. The prosthetic valve and sternal sutures may be visible.

3.1.1.2 Global Cardiomegaly

Long-standing cardiac failure may result in global cardiac enlargement (Fig. 3.3).

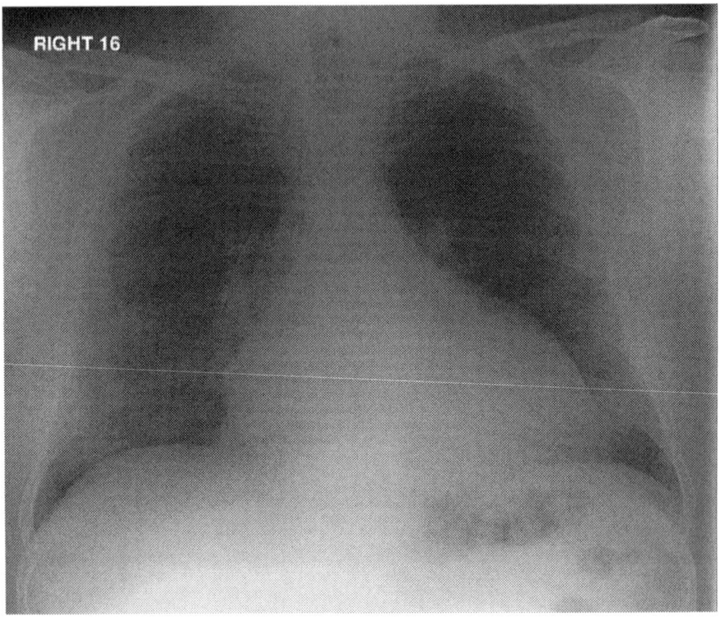

FIGURE 3.3. Global cardiomegaly.

3.1.1.3 Pericardial Effusion

A pericardial effusion typically produces a globular-shaped heart and the cardiac border may be better defined as cardiac motion is reduced (Fig. 3.4). The alteration in heart shape may be more noticeable in comparison with previous imaging.

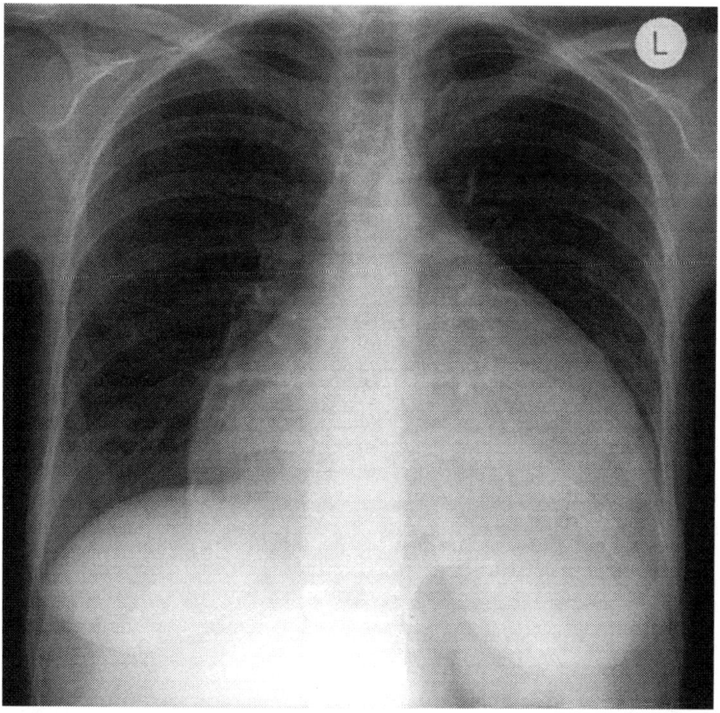

FIGURE 3.4. Pericardial effusion.

3.1.1.4 Pulmonary Hypertension

Figure 3.5 shows marked enlargement of the pulmonary arteries and pulmonary plethora as a result of untreated atrial septal defect.

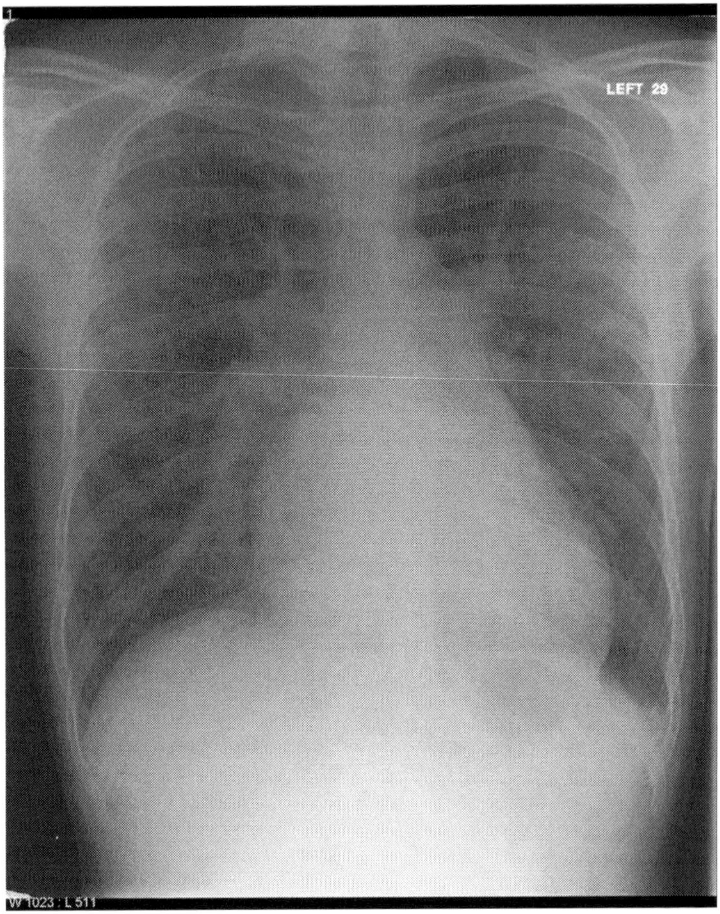

FIGURE 3.5. Pulmonary hypertension in a patient with an untreated atrial septal defect.

3.1.1.5 Ventricular Aneurysm

Aneurysmal dilatation of the ventricle may occur postinfarction. This shows as a focal bulge of the left heart border with high-density calcification in its rim (Fig. 3.6). This may be present on previous films.

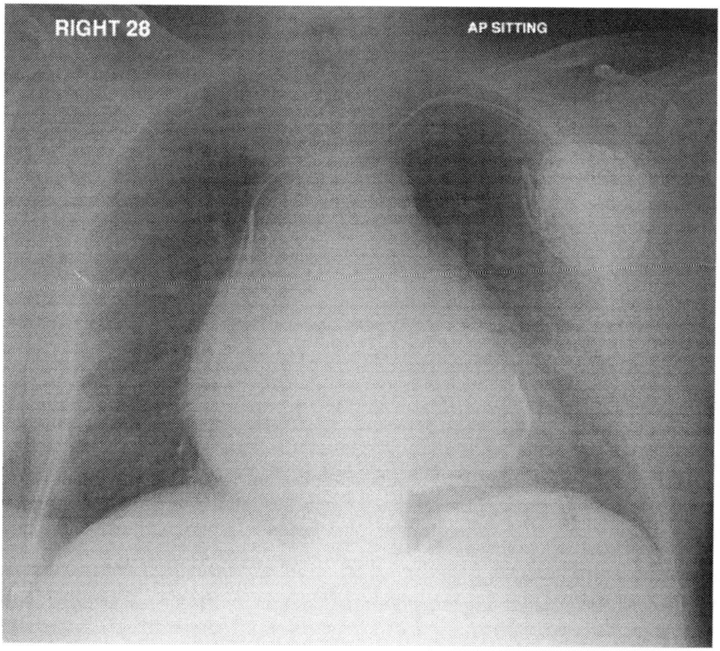

FIGURE 3.6. Calcified ventricular aneurysm.

Other causes of alteration of the cardiac contour include surgery such as cardiac transplantation (Fig. 3.7) and congenital variation, for example, dextrocardia (Fig. 3.8) and right-sided aortic arch (Fig. 3.9).

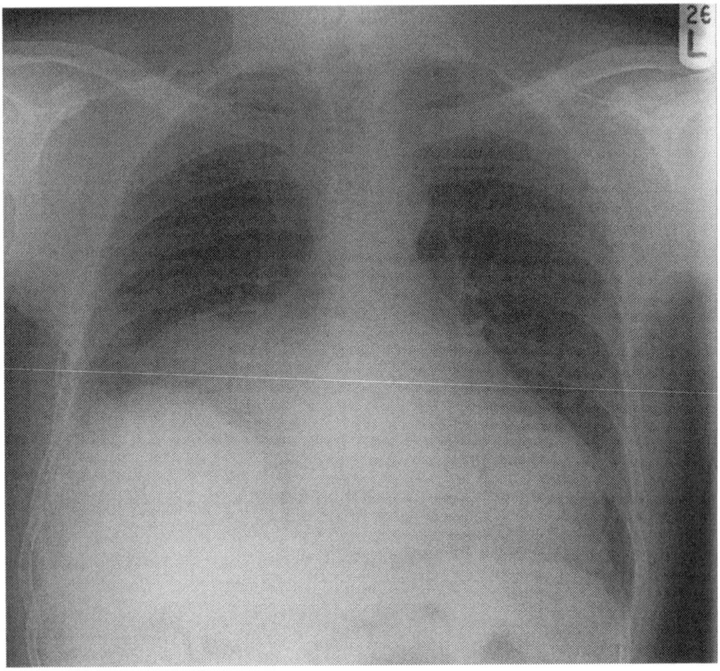

FIGURE 3.7. Cardiac transplant, the native heart is in situ and the transplanted heart gives an extra right-sided bulge.

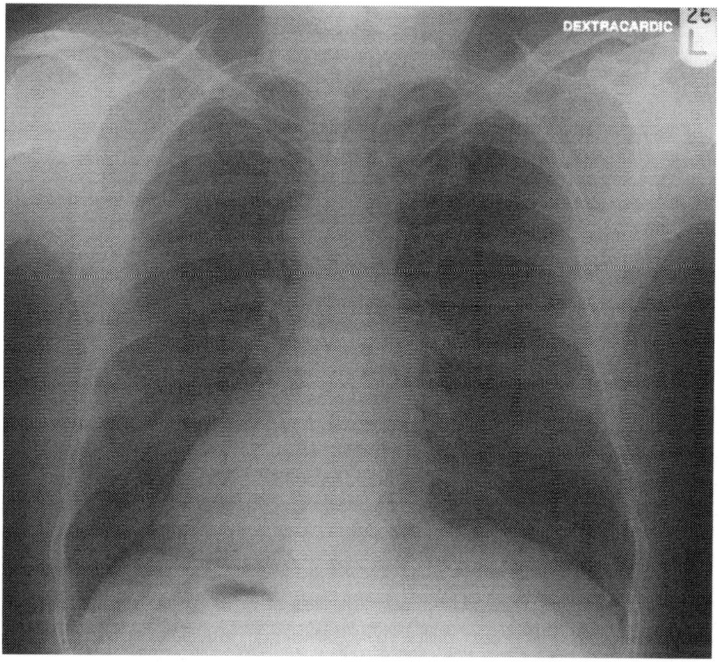

FIGURE 3.8. Dextrocardia in this case with situs inversus, note right-sided stomach bubble.

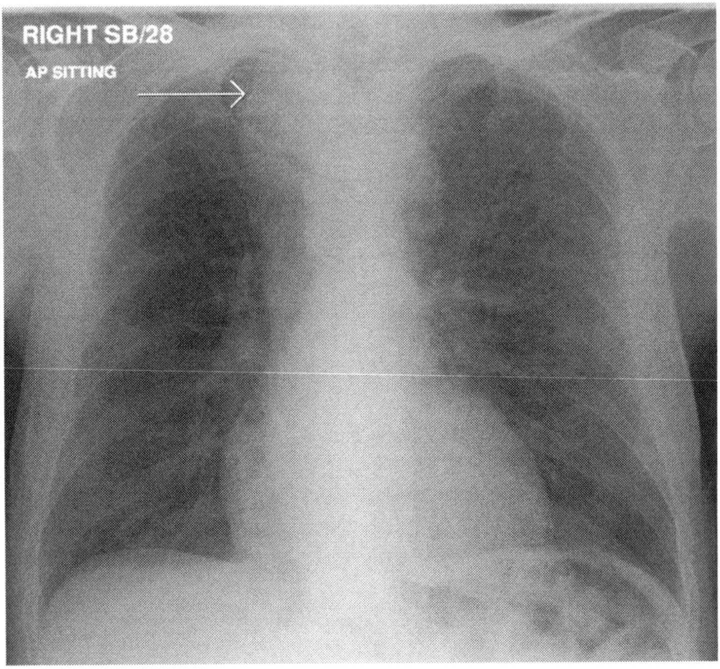

FIGURE 3.9. Right-sided aortic arch seen as a well-defined structure within the right paratracheal space (*arrow*).

3.1.2 Hilar Abnormalities

3.1.2.1 Unilateral Hilar Mass

The appearance of the hilar regions should be roughly symmetrical. Asymmetry may indicate a focal mass. A relatively tapering appearance to the abnormality is suggestive of a vascular origin, which includes conditions such as a unilateral pulmonary artery aneurysm.

Loss of clarity of the hilar bay or angle is much more suggestive of a soft tissue abnormality, including enlargement of lymph nodes. Unilateral lymph node enlargement can be caused by primary tuberculosis. Asymmetrical lymph node enlargement occurs in lymphoma, but it is important to exclude nodal disease secondary to an underlying lung

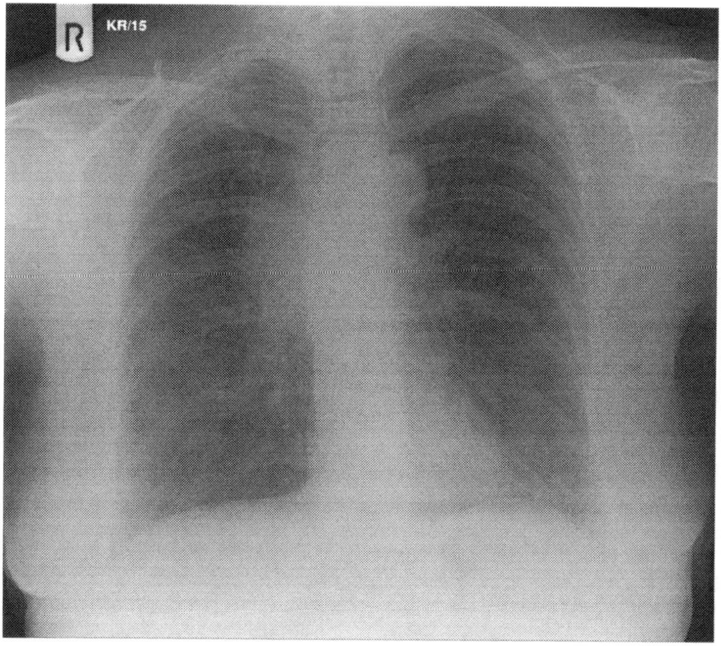

FIGURE 3.10. Unilateral hilar mass.

neoplasm. The soft tissue density at the hilum may itself represent a primary bronchogenic carcinoma (Fig. 3.10).

In general a computed tomography (CT) scan is likely to be required for further evaluation.

3.1.2.2 Bilateral Hilar Lymph Node Enlargement

It can occasionally be difficult to differentiate between large hilar lymph nodes, enlarged pulmonary arteries, or simply a prominence of the hilar region. Lymph nodes tend to be more radiodense than vessels and loss of the hilar bay is a good indication of lymph nodes (Fig. 3.11). Vessels can often be traced more distally and are generally of a tapering appearance. Occasionally if the initial film was performed AP, a repeat film in a PA projection can be helpful, and comparison with old films is often useful. Again if uncertainty persists, a CT scan will help.

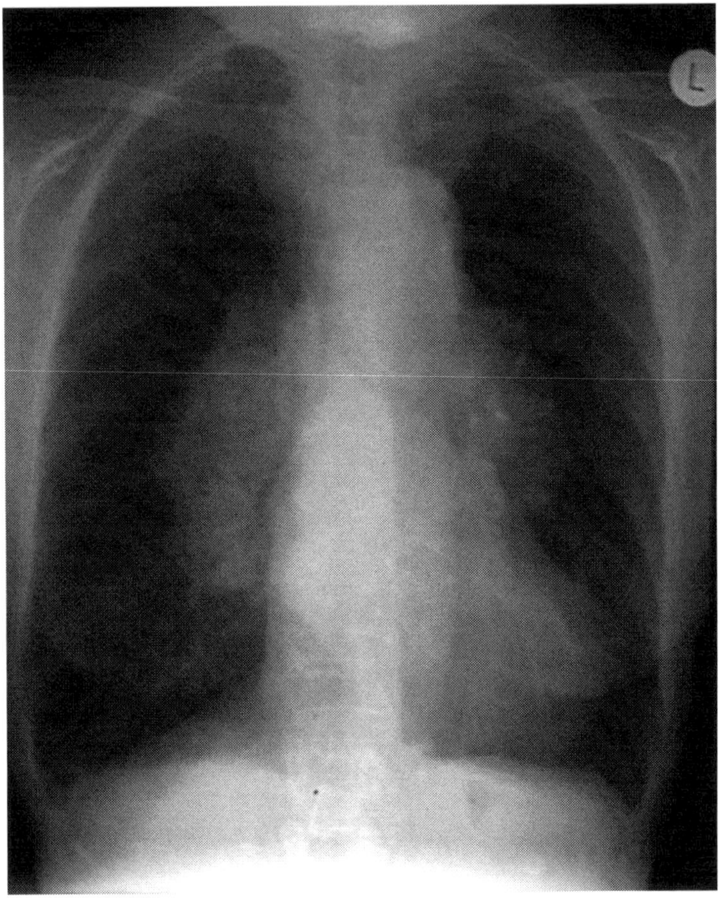

FIGURE 3.11. Bilateral hilar lymphadenopathy.

While bilateral hilar lymph node enlargement is a classical feature of sarcoidosis, other conditions such as lymphoma and metastatic disease will need to be considered.

3.1.3 Other Middle Mediastinal Abnormalities

3.1.3.1 Pneumomediastinum

Pneumomediastinum is a result of air being forced into the soft tissues. Common causes include acute asthma, pushing in childbirth, straining at stool, and voluntary valsalva maneuver, which occurs when taking various illicit drugs, such as Ecstasy.

Pneumomediastinum may also be traumatic; this may be external trauma such as stabbing or RTA, or iatrogenic post-dilatation of a strictured oesophagus.

The pericardium is not normally seen on a chest X-ray. If it is separated from the myocardium by air, this will establish a new soft tissue interface and the margins will be seen (Fig. 3.12a). Similarly air tracking into the mediastinum will alter the sharp margination and will give a slightly shaggy ill-defined appearance (Fig. 3.12b). This may also be accompanied by subcutaneous emphysema.

FIGURE 3.12. (a) Pneumomediastinum showing air tracking along mediastinum (*arrows*), (b) pneumomediastinum showing shaggy ill-defined appearance of mediastinum and lifting of pericardium (*arrow*).

a
b

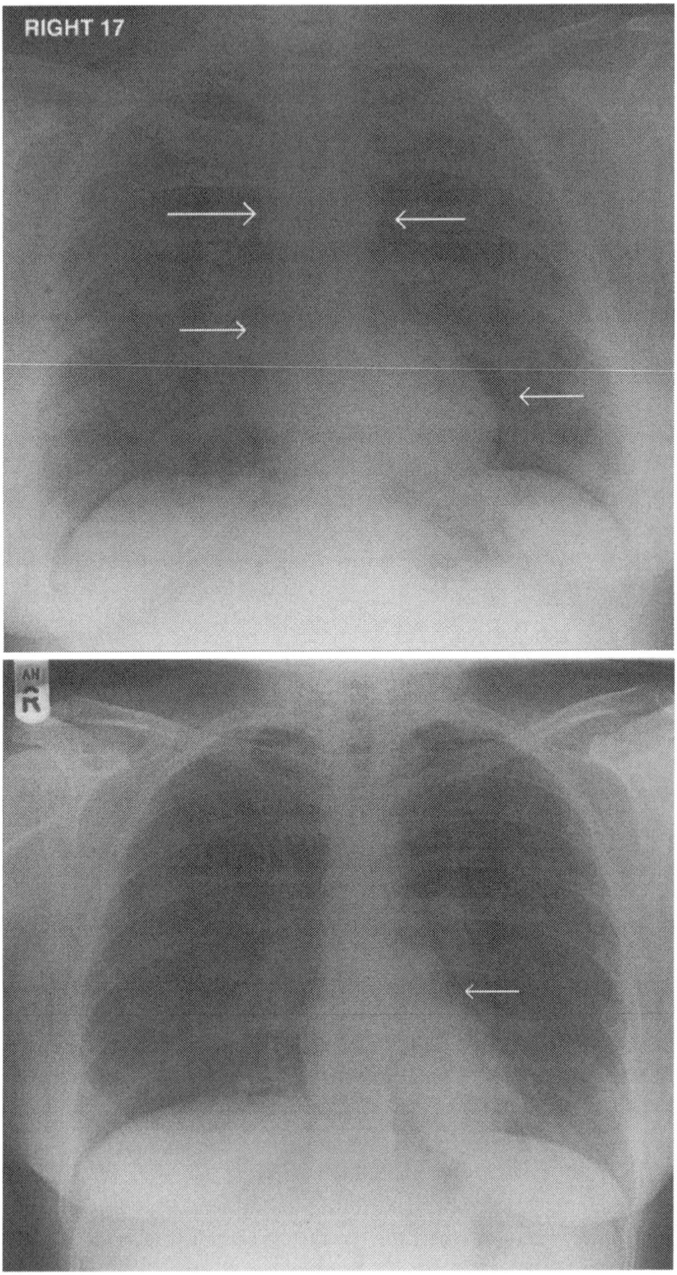

FIGURE 3.12. (continued).

3.1.3.2 Pericardial Fat Pad

Loss of clarity of the cardiophrenic angle may result from a pericardial fat pad. This is often inseparable from the mediastinum, but should be of relatively lower density, being made up of fat, rather than muscle (Fig. 3.13). The heart border should be preserved. It is often also present on previous imaging.

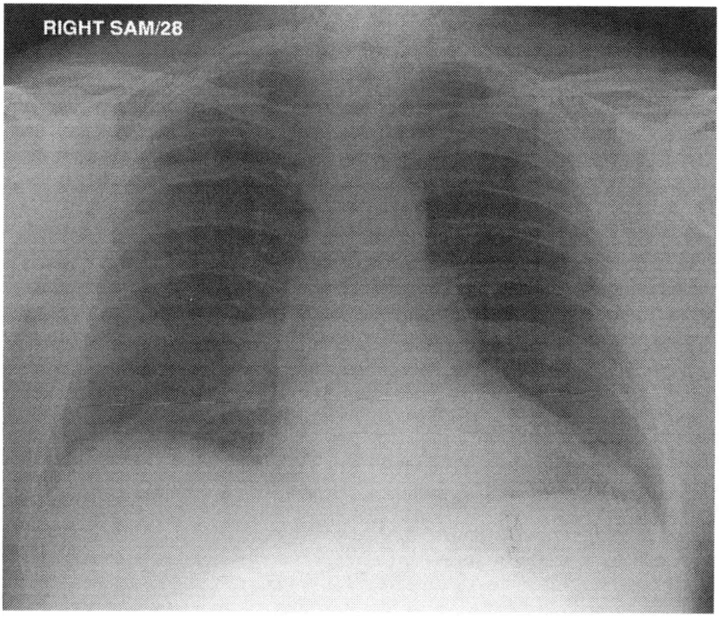

FIGURE 3.13. Left-sided pericardial fat pad.

3.1.3.3 Pectus Excavatum

The chest wall shape created by pectus excavatum will alter how the mediastinal contour projects. There is loss of the right heart border and the anterior ribs generally appear more vertical than usual (Fig. 3.14). The abnormality itself should be obvious on examining the patient.

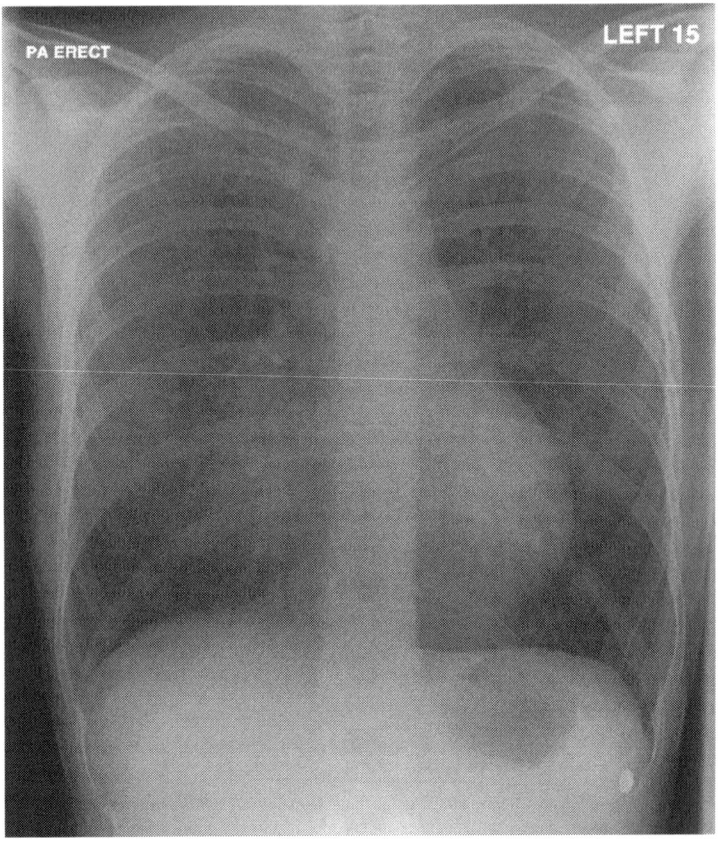

FIGURE 3.14. Pectus excavatum.

3.2 Anterior Mediastinum

The location of a mediastinal abnormality can be worked out by its effect on other adjacent structures. If there is a loss of clarity of an anterior mediastinal structure and preservation of middle and posterior mediastinal structures, the abnormality must lie within the anterior mediastinum. Similarly, if there is deviation or compression of the trachea within the superior mediastinum, the abnormality must lie within the anterior superior mediastinum.

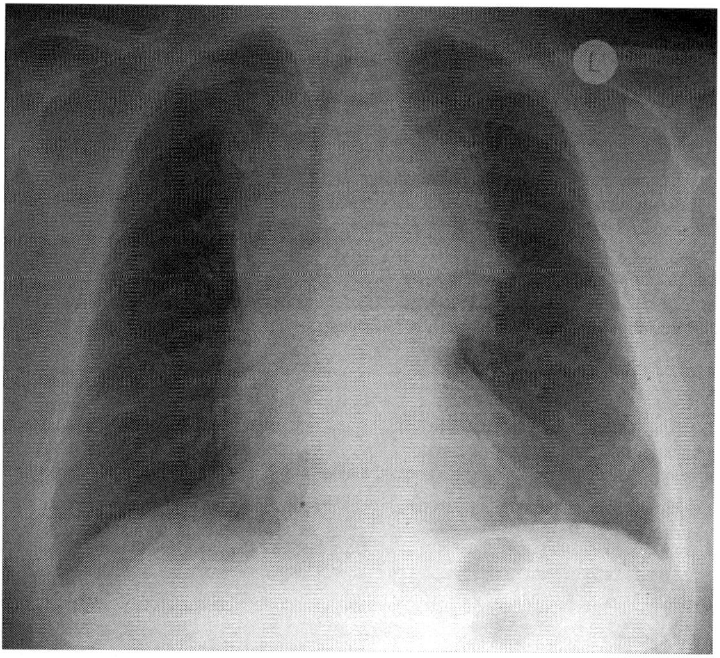

FIGURE 3.15. Anterior mediastinal mass in a patient with a teratoma.

Remember that the descending aorta is a posterior mediastinal structure and preservation of this soft tissue air interface suggests that abnormalities seen are not in the posterior mediastinum.

The commonest causes for anterior mediastinal abnormalities are thyroid masses, thymomas, teratodermoids, and enlargement of lymph nodes typically in lymphoma (Fig. 3.15). This is most commonly remembered as being the four T's (lymphoma being described as "terrible" lymphoma). Any of these masses could be malignant.

In the example given there is deviation and narrowing of the trachea with preservation of the aortic contour (Fig. 3.15).

3.3 Posterior Mediastinum

Abnormalities within the posterior mediastinum will cause loss of outline of other posterior mediastinal structures, for example, the descending thoracic aorta, oesophagus, or spine.

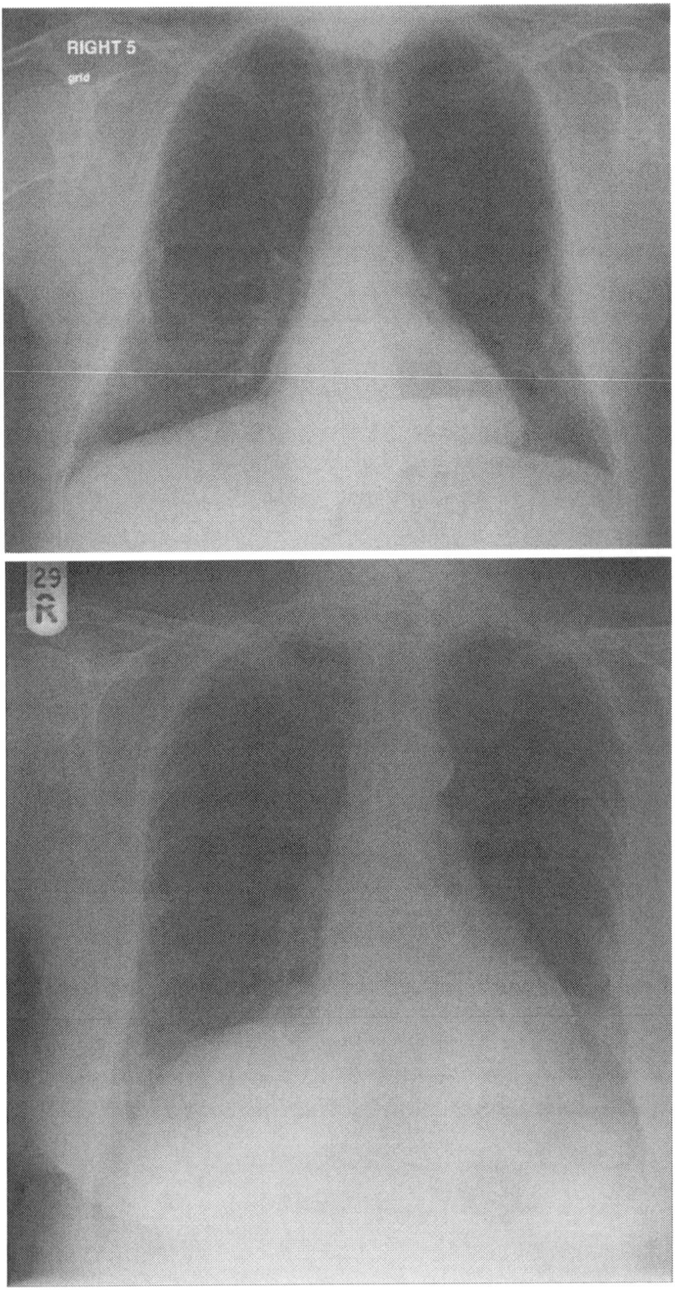

FIGURE 3.16. (a) Hiatus hernia showing air fluid level within stomach. (b) Hiatus hernia shown passing through diaphragm.

3.3.1 Hiatus Hernia

A hiatus hernia will project as a mass behind the heart. Clues to its true nature are the presence of the fluid level (Fig. 3.16a) and absence of the normal stomach bubble beneath the diaphragm. Often a stomach-shaped density is simply seen behind the heart (Fig. 3.16b). Once again this abnormality is frequently seen on previous films.

3.3.2 Gastric Pull Through Following Oesophagectomy

The appearances are similar to a hiatus hernia, but the air-filled dilated structure passes more superiorly and reaches the superior mediastinum (Fig. 3.17). Surgical clips are often seen.

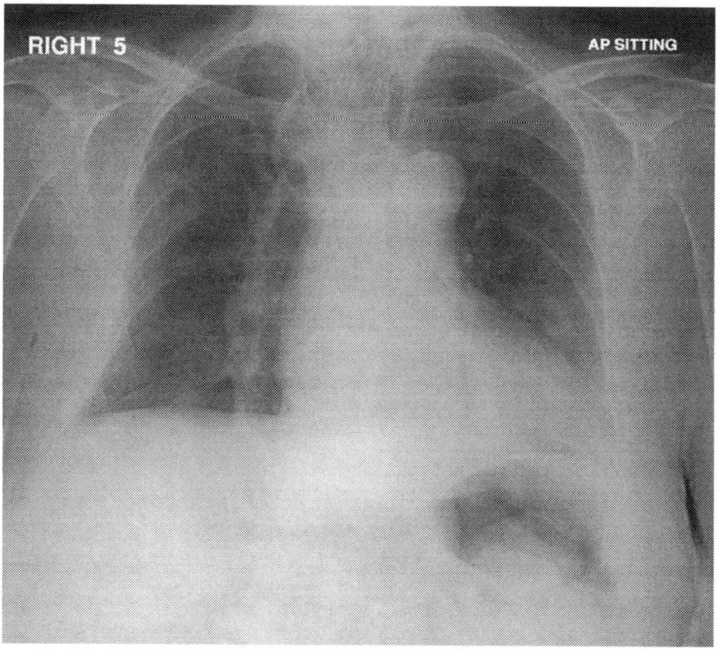

FIGURE 3.17. Gastric pull through showing air-filled structure within superior mediastinum.

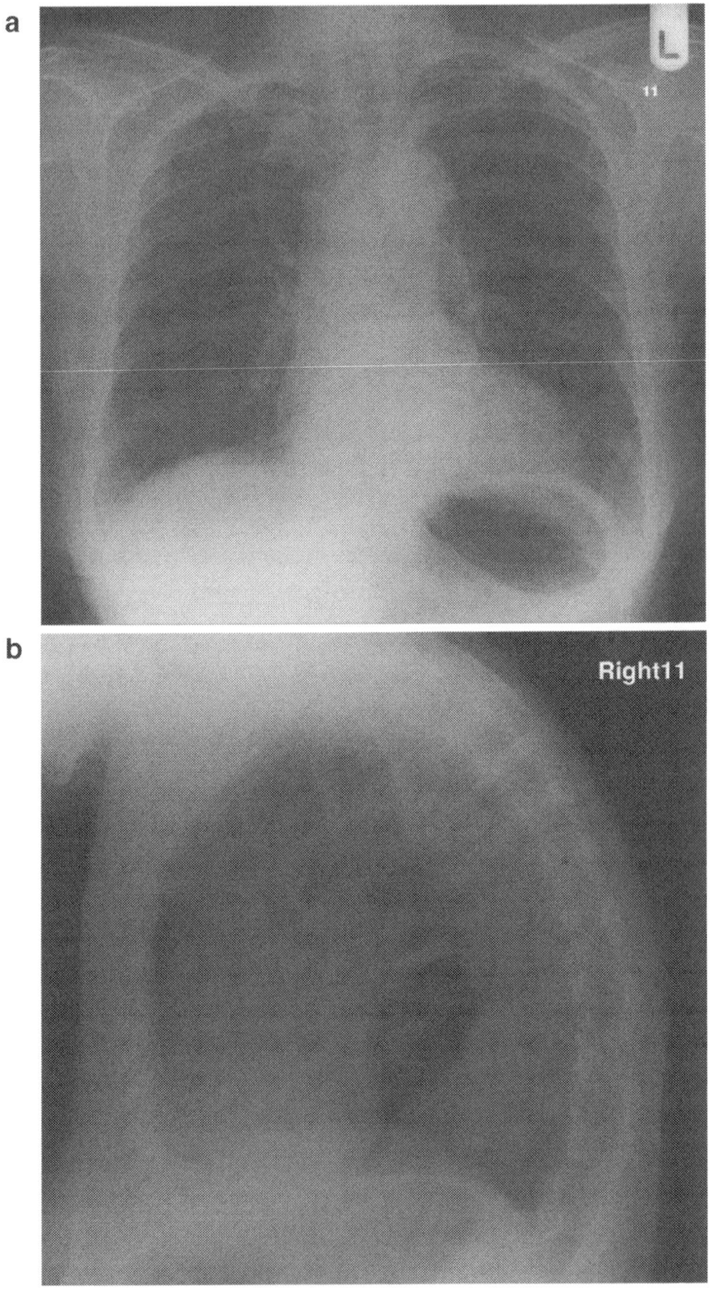

FIGURE 3.18. Oesophageal dilatation: (a) PA and (b) lateral views showing air-filled dilated Oesophagus in a patient with achalasia.

3.3.3 Oesophageal Dilatation

Causes of oesophageal dilatation include primary oesophageal carcinoma and, as in the example below, achalasia (Fig. 3.18a). Again an air-filled structure is seen extending into the superior mediastinum. The oesophagus is a posterior structure clearly seen on the lateral view (Fig. 3.18b).

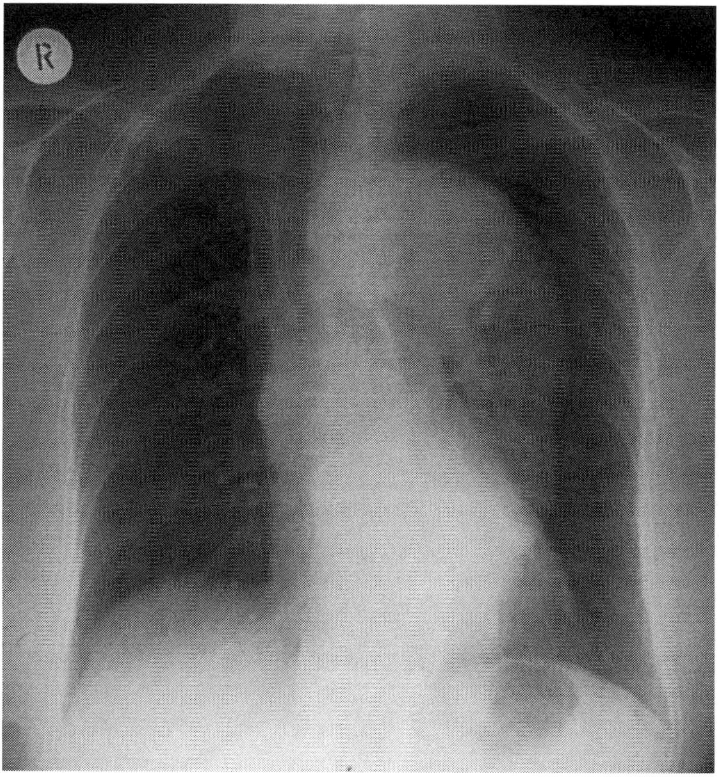

FIGURE 3.19. Descending thoracic aortic aneurysm.

3.3.4 Descending Thoracic Aortic Abnormalities

The normal contour of the descending thoracic aorta will be lost and curvilinear opacity extending from the hemithorax is often seen (Fig. 3.19).

The anterior and middle mediastinal structures will be maintained, so for example, the left heart border and hilar regions will project normally.

Signs of a ruptured thoracic aortic aneurysm can be seen on plain films. These include a left apical cap, which is an effusion (blood) seen at the apex on a supine film.

3.4 Key Points

1) The mediastinum consists of anterior, middle, and posterior regions.
2) Any abnormality will alter the outline of its own compartment, with preservation of the outline of the remaining compartments.

Chapter 4
Basic Patterns of Lung Disease

Introduction

This chapter aims to give the reader confidence in diagnosing the various abnormalities that occur within the lungs by providing a structured approach to interpretation. It is, therefore, divided into subsections relating to the various basic patterns of abnormality that diseases of the lungs produce on chest X-ray. This includes consolidation, reticular change (lines), and nodules among others.

As with much of the practice of medicine, things are not always straightforward and patients may have more than one pathology demonstrated on their chest X-ray.

Multiple pathologies may be related, such as a pulmonary mass with evidence of lymphangitis. They may not necessarily be related, but be equally important to consider in terms of treatment, for example, pulmonary fibrosis with consolidation. Equally while there may be multiple abnormalities on a chest X-ray, one may predominate and be the dominant diagnosis.

It is therefore important to recognize what is the predominant pattern of abnormality. For example, the main abnormality may be linear, such as reticulation in the bases or perihilar regions found in left ventricular failure. It may be multiple tiny nodules, such as miliary tuberculosis. In each of these cases the background "appearance" of the lungs may not be

R. Joarder, N. Crundwell (eds.), *Chest X-Ray in Clinical Practice*,
DOI 10.1007/978-1-84882-099-9_4,

normal and there may be other abnormalities to be found, for example, underlying lung emphysema.

With time, practice, and experience, it is possible to pick out the predominant pattern quickly. Initially, however, it is very important to make a deliberate effort to identify which patterns are seen and then decide which is predominant. Having done this, a sensible list of diagnoses can be generated.

Within the following chapters we introduce the basic radiological patterns created by lung disease, giving examples of common or typical findings.

Chapter 4a
Consolidation

Consolidation is a commonly found abnormality on a chest X-ray and its correct interpretation is of relevance to the patient. The term consolidation is often misused and its appearance is often misinterpreted. In order to understand what consolidation actually represents, it is important to have a good understanding of the basic lung anatomy, in particular of the smaller structures that make up the lungs.

Consolidation is the presence of a substance within the alveoli that displaces normal air (Fig. 4.1a and b). This results in a relative increase in radio-density of the affected area.

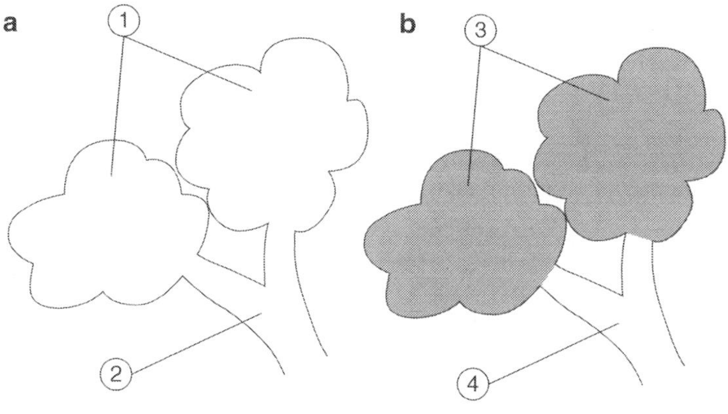

FIGURE 4.1. Diagrams to show (a) normal alveoli and bronchioles; (b) consolidation with material, e.g., pus-filled alveolus with sparing of the bronchiole which remains air filled. (1) Air-filled alveoli; (2) air-filled bronchioles; (3) pus-filled alveoli (consolidation); (4) air-filled bronchioles.

TABLE 4.1. Five major categories of substances that result in consolidation.

Fluid: cardiac failure, near drowning
Cellular material: pus in infection, malignant cells in alveolar cell carcinoma
Aspirated material : vomitus
Proteinaceous material : alveolar proteinosis
Blood: pulmonary haemorrhage

There are major categories of substance that result in such displacement.

These are fluid, cellular material (inflammatory or malignant cells), aspirated material, proteinaceous material, and blood (see Table 4.1).

Consolidation is also sometimes referred to as alveolar opacification or air space opacity.

Remember that we identify structures on a radiograph due to the interface between materials of different density. We therefore do not normally see air within the peripheral airways or air spaces as separate entities, as the airways are full of air adjacent to air-filled alveoli. Once there is consolidation within the alveoli, this displaces the air leaving adjacent branching airways that remain air filled. As the air-filled airways are up against material-filled alveoli, we are now able to see them as independent branching structures. These are termed "air bronchograms" (Fig. 4.2).

Air bronchograms are not always present, but if they are, they are very helpful in the correct identification of consolidation.

Other features that will help you decide whether the "white blobs" you see are consolidation or another abnormality such as a mass include

a) Ill-defined opacity/opacities that may coalesce
b) Opacities that conform to the approximate shape of a lobe as in lobar pneumonia (typically pneumococcus)

The location of the consolidation may help in establishing a diagnosis. For example, perihilar consolidation tends to

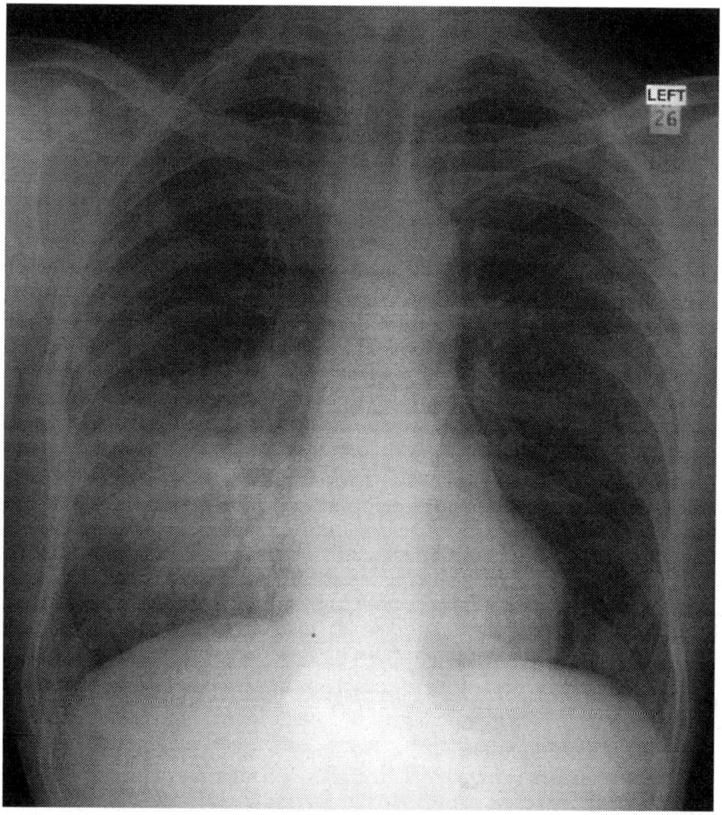

FIGURE 4.2. Right middle lobe consolidation with air bronchograms.

occur more in atypical infections and is also associated with left ventricular failure. Consolidation may be multi-focal, for example, in sarcoidosis, and multi-focal consolidation that alters its location over a period of time occurs in eosinophilic pneumonias.

As you may have gathered consolidation (air space opacity) is a rather non-specific finding and can represent the effect of a large number of pathological processes. Having identified air space opacity, it is important to review the remaining film to see if there are any ancillary features that would help in establishing the underlying cause. These may include an enlarged cardiothoracic ratio and peripheral septal lines in pulmonary edema, a more lobar distribution in a pneumonic process, and so on.

As a general rule serial imaging should be obtained to ensure resolution. Remember that radiological clearance may lag behind clinical improvement.

4.1 Examples of Consolidation and Its Causes

4.1.1 Infection

There is opacification within the lower zone of the right lung. Air bronchograms may be present. In the given example there is loss of definition of the right heart border (Fig. 4.3a, b). From this you can work out where the consolidation is located. The right middle lobe (which is normally air filled) is adjacent to the right atrium. This is why you normally see the margin of the right atrium. The consolidation within the right middle lobe causes loss of the air/soft tissue interface and hence loss of definition of the border.

From the image itself it is not possible categorically to say that this is due to infection. However, the focal unilateral appearance, combined with clinical history such as a relatively rapid onset of abnormality with cough and pyrexia, would make infection the most likely diagnosis.

In Fig. 4.4 there is consolidation and air bronchograms are present. In this example there is loss of the left heart border. The lingular segment of the left upper lobe lies adjacent to the left heart border. When consolidation occurs the air/soft tissue interface is lost so the left heart border is lost.

a
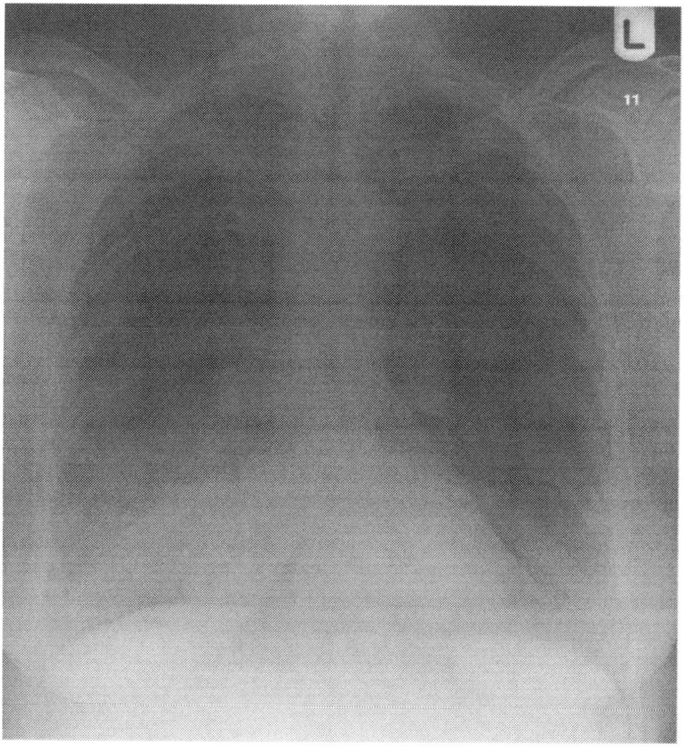

FIGURE 4.3. (continued).

b

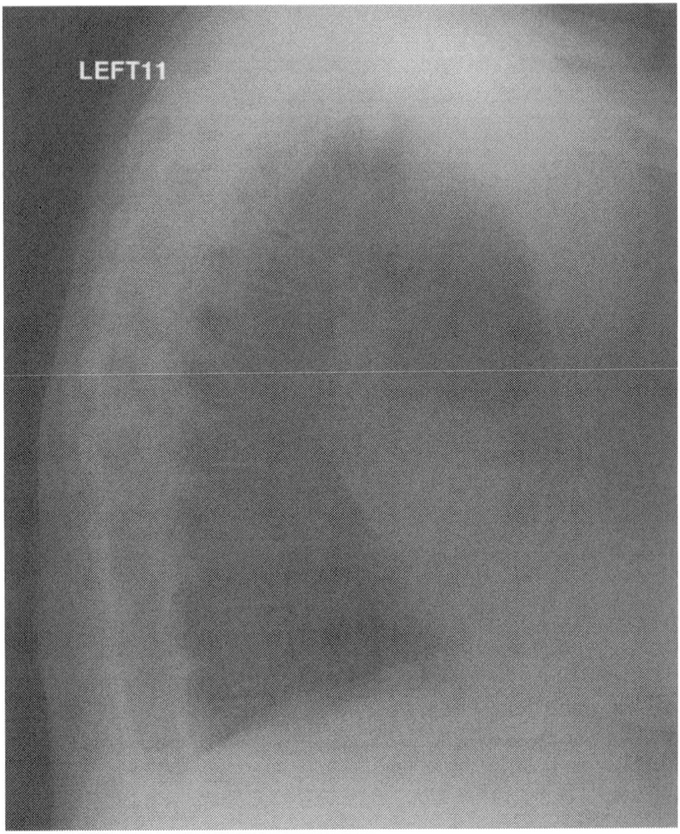

FIGURE 4.3. (a) PA and (b) lateral views of right middle lobe consolidation.

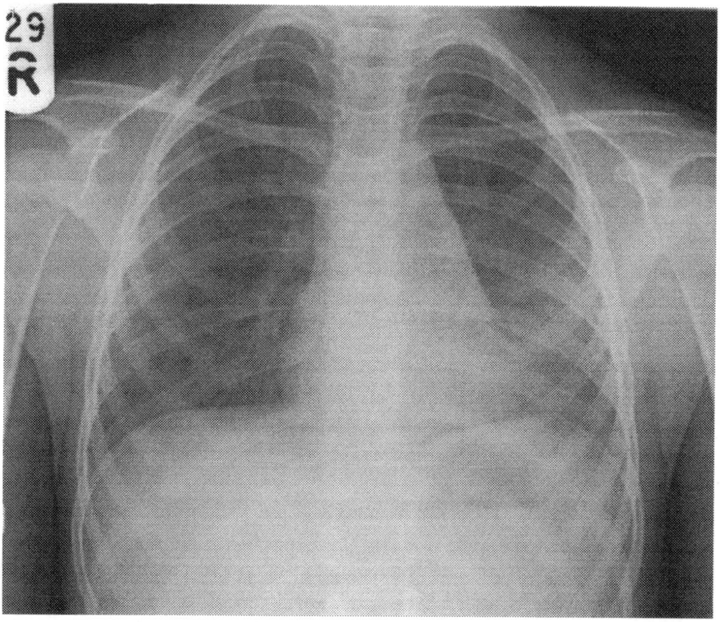

FIGURE 4.4. Lingular consolidation.

4.1.2 Pulmonary Oedema

The changes of pulmonary oedema are not purely those of consolidation. In the early stages there may be ground glass opacity seen in a perihilar distribution. This is a reflection of fluid filling the alveolar spaces.

Ground glass opacity is defined as a diffuse increase in opacity which on plain film results in the loss of the vascular pattern.

Once there is sufficient fluid within the alveoli, particularly adjacent alveoli, then a more typical pattern of air space opacity is seen (Fig. 4.5). In addition to this linear abnormality is seen. This is due to thickening of the inter-lobular septa or septal lines, also known as Kerley's lines. These will be described in more detail in Chapter 4c.

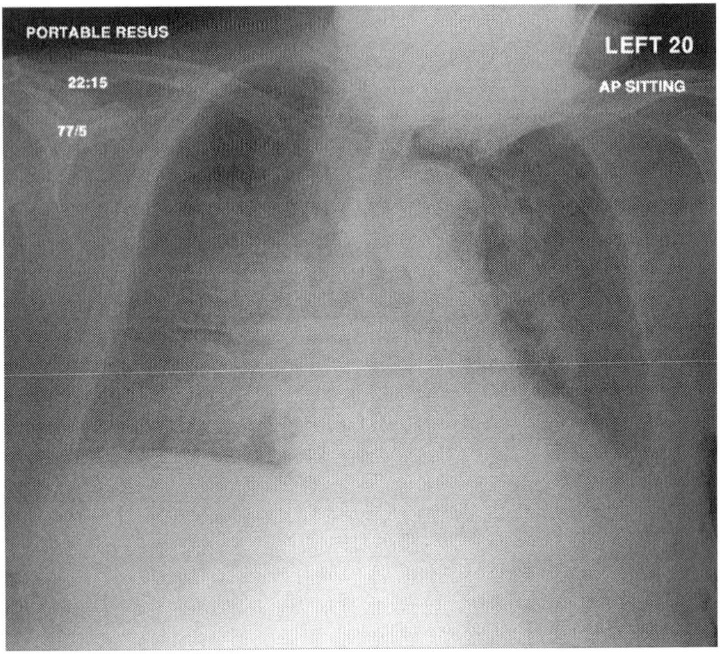

FIGURE 4.5. Pulmonary oedema.

When interpreting the appearance of consolidation, correlation with the clinical findings is important. Remember that the differential diagnosis of air space opacity is very broad, but a pattern of perihilar and basal ground glass opacity with consolidation, peripheral septal markings, and pleural effusion is very suggestive of pulmonary oedema.

4.1.3 Malignancy

In alveolar cell carcinoma there is often a gradual development of pure consolidation (Fig. 4.6). There may be weight loss, but without accompanying clinical features of infection. The condition is often unilateral and focal, but can be multifocal. Lymphoma may also appear as consolidation.

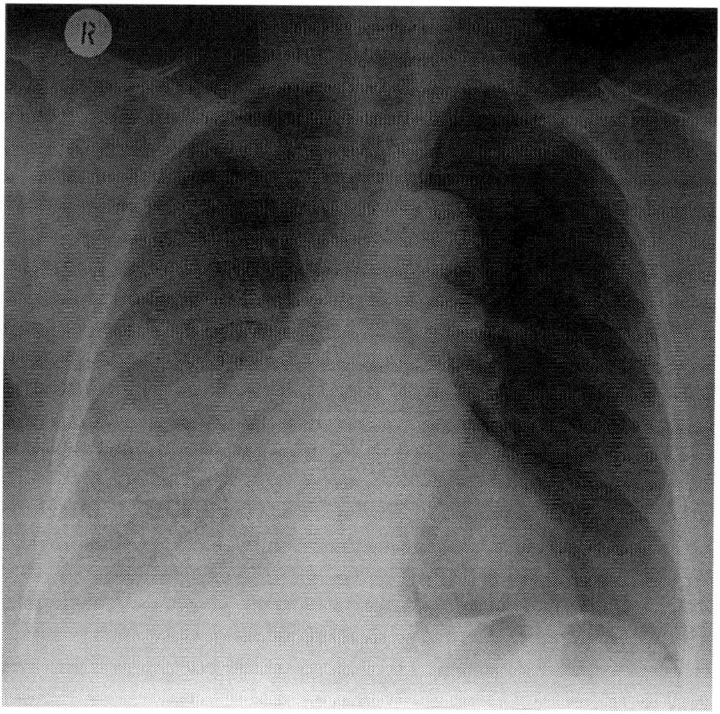

FIGURE 4.6. Alveolar cell carcinoma.

4.1.4 Haemorrhage

Blood in the alveolar spaces displaces air resulting in air space opacity. It may also have a slightly more ground glass appearance (Fig. 4.7) and can be very extensive. Once again the findings are non-specific, but the diagnosis may be suggested by the patient's underlying condition or a history of haemoptysis. This is most often found in patients who are generally unwell, in particular the HDU/ITU setting. There is also a tendency to pulmonary haemorrhage in connective tissue diseases, for example, scleroderma.

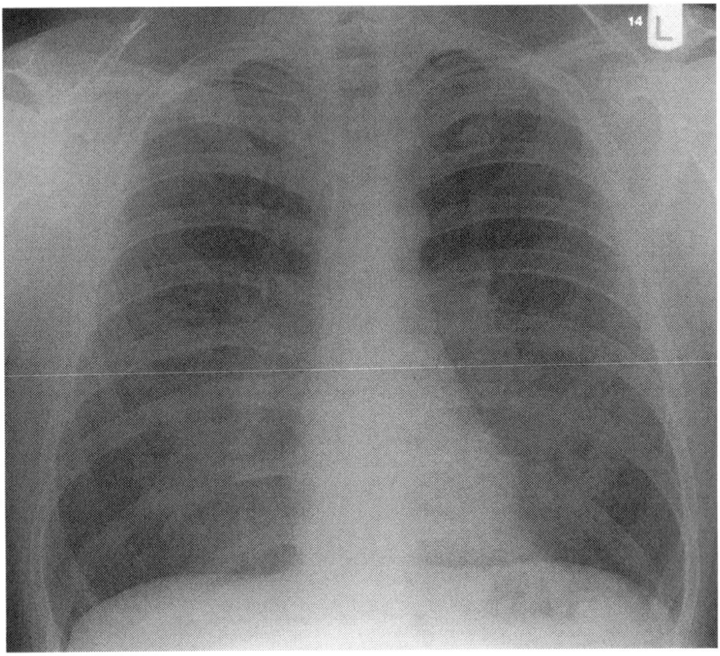

FIGURE 4.7. Pulmonary haemorrhage appearing as ground glass opacity bibasally.

4.2 Key Points

1) Consolidation is a non-specific finding.
2) The pattern and ancillary features may suggest the cause.
3) Follow-up to ensure resolution is important.
4) Radiological clearance can lag behind clinical improvement.

Chapter 4b
Collapse

Collapse can involve an individual lobe, several lobes, or the whole of one lung. Remember that the right lung has three lobes and the left lung has two. Collapse may also be segmental or sub-segmental within a lobe. These latter types of collapse are dealt with in a subsequent chapter, as the abnormalities they produce radiologically tend to be linear.

Collapse can be due to obstruction of the airway by material within the airway, material within the wall, or material outside the airway (Table 4.2).

TABLE 4.2. Causes of airway obstruction.

Material within the airway (airway obstruction)
Malignancy
Foreign body
Mucus plugging
Material outside the airway (extrinsic compression)
Fluid, e.g., pleural effusion
Air, e.g., pneumothorax
Extrinsic mass

4.3 Lobar Collapse

When a lobe collapses it is no longer filled with air. Therefore, its radiodensity will increase. The amount of space it occupies is reduced, causing "volume loss." Volume loss is an important and sometimes subtle, but often overlooked, sign on a chest X-ray. The loss of volume caused by the collapse of the lobe may result in other anatomical structures moving into the space previously occupied by the lung. Examples include movement of the lung fissures, shift of the mediastinum, relative crowding of the ribs, and elevation of the hemi-diaphragm.

When collapsed, each of the five lobes produces an appearance that is typical. These appearances result from their relationships to surrounding structures and loss of existing soft tissue interfaces or creation of new ones.

4.4 Right Lung

In general it is easier to see the radiological changes of collapse of the lobes of the right lung, but the effects of the volume loss is often more subtle, as the lobes themselves are smaller.

Right upper lobe collapse is generally easy to see on a chest X-ray. There is a dense infilling of the right upper zone above

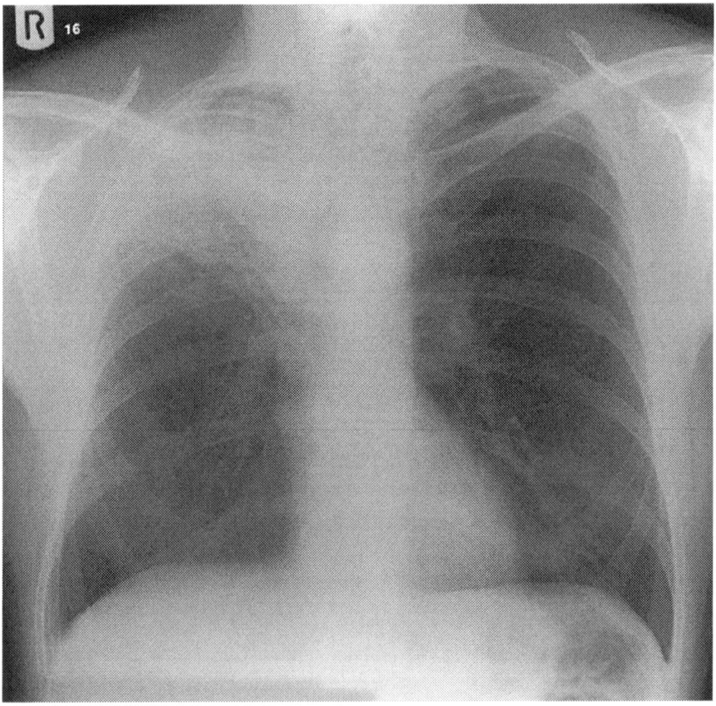

FIGURE 4.8. Right upper lobe collapse.

the horizontal fissure which is pulled upward (Fig. 4.8). If there is no movement of the horizontal fissure it is more likely that the appearances represent consolidation within the right upper lobe.

The right lower lobe is in contact with the right hemi-diaphragm. A collapse therefore produces a dense opacity within the right base and loss of the outline of the right hemi-diaphragm. In addition there is loss of volume within the right base. In the example given there is obscuration of the medial aspect of the right hemi-diaphragm with preservation of the right heart border (Fig. 4.9).

The right middle lobe is in contact with the right heart border and therefore collapse removes this soft tissue interface, causing loss of the outline of the right heart border (Fig. 4.10). Dense opacity is seen within the right base and again there is volume loss.

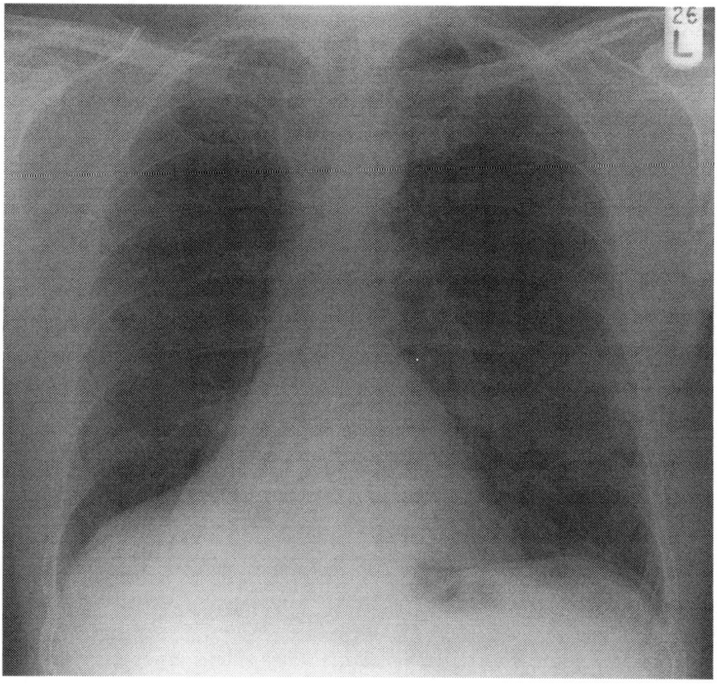

FIGURE 4.9. Right lower lobe collapse.

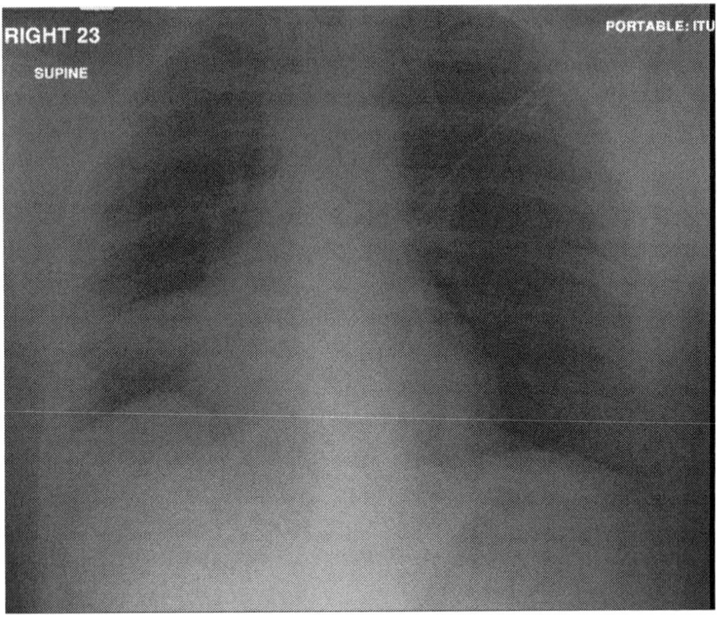

FIGURE 4.10. Right middle lobe collapse.

4.5 Left Lung

Collapse of the lobes of the left lung causes more subtle radiological abnormalities and these can be difficult to pick up. They do, however, reflect the basic principles of X-ray interpretation and are caused by the altered relationships with the adjacent structures. If you remember why they occur and you look for them, you will be much less likely to overlook or misinterpret them.

The left lower lobe is in contact with the left hemi-diaphragm. When it collapses it does so in a medial and inferior direction, to end up posterior to the heart (Fig. 4.11). This creates a triangular-shaped dense opacity that projects behind the left side of the heart, the so-called "sail sign." In addition there is loss of the air–soft tissue interface of the medial aspect of the left hemi-diaphragm and this portion of the

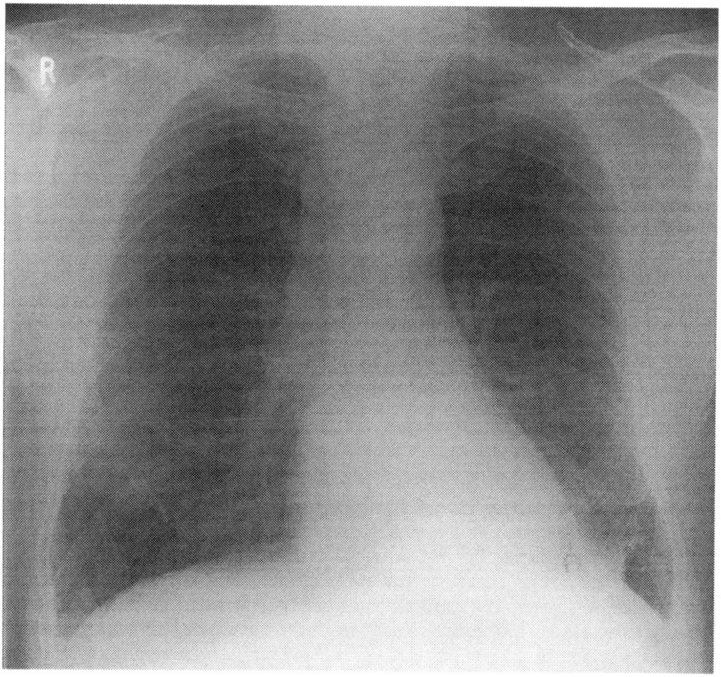

FIGURE 4.11. Left lower lobe collapse.

hemi-diaphragm is no longer visualized. There may be signs of volume loss, such as inferior movement of the hilar region.

Left upper lobe collapse is probably the most difficult lobar collapse to identify radiologically and is the one that is most often misinterpreted.

Remember that the left upper lobe extends from the apex to the left cardiac border, the latter being in contact with the lingular segment. Collapse of the lobe produces a veil-like opacity over the entire hemi-thorax, particularly the more superior portion. The outline of the aortic knuckle is often preserved or may be enhanced because this region becomes adjacent to aerated left lower lobe. The soft tissue interface is maintained, creating the so-called "Luftsichel" sign (air scythe) (Fig. 4.12). Further evidence of collapse is suggested by volume loss, particularly crowding of the lateral ribs and elevation of the left hemi-diaphragm.

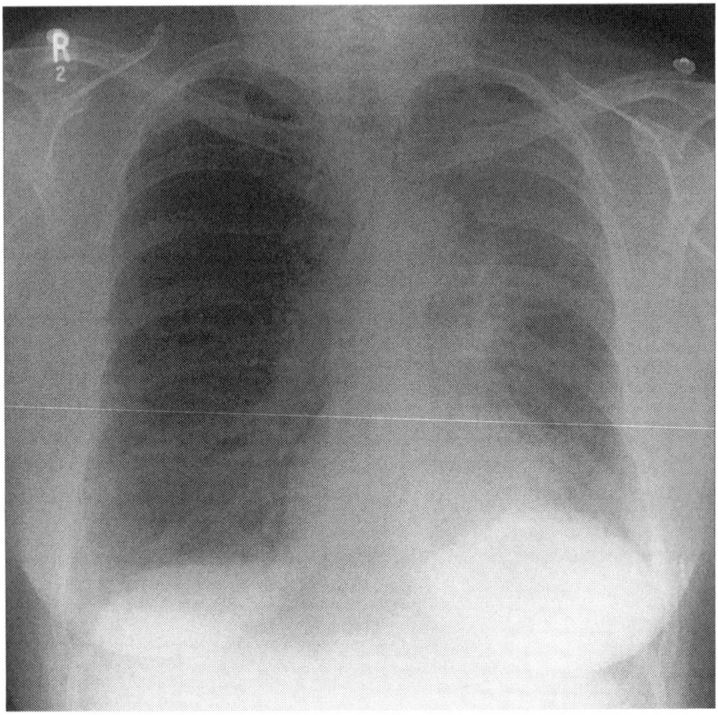

FIGURE 4.12. Left upper lobe collapse. Note air crescent around aorta "Luftsichel" sign.

Left upper lobe collapse is often associated with an obstructing carcinoma situated at the left hilum. This may be visible on the chest X-ray, as it is in the example given here.

4.6 Whole Lung Collapse

There is complete loss of air within the hemi-thorax resulting in complete opacification, "a white out." Note that there is mediastinal shift toward the side of the collapse (Fig. 4.13). A large pleural effusion would also create a complete white out. The two can be differentiated by the positioning of the mediastinum. A pleural effusion will exert mass effect and push the mediastinum away from it, whereas collapse pulls the mediastinum toward it. It is also important to differentiate acutely

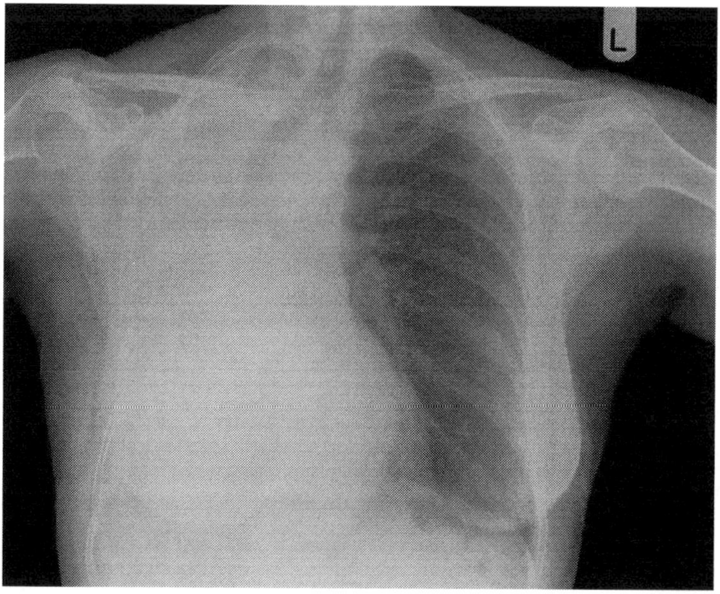

FIGURE 4.13. Complete collapse of the right lung.

collapsed lung from lung volume loss caused by pneumonectomy. There is likely to be evidence of previous surgery on chest X-ray and metallic clips, rib abnormality, etc. There is also usually a history from the patient or notes. Findings may also be confirmed in comparison with the previous film.

4.7 Key Points

1) Volume loss is an important sign of collapse.
2) Displacement of normal structures is an indication of volume loss.
3) Collapse alters the normal air–soft tissue interface.
4) The five lobes have specific patterns associated with their collapse.
5) Follow-up to ensure resolution is important.

Chapter 4c
Lines

The chest X-ray that you are interpreting will often have more than one type of abnormality present. It is therefore important to decide what is the predominant type or pattern of abnormality that you are seeing. If the abnormality seen is predominantly linear, a reticular pattern, then the pathologies within this chapter will need to be considered Table 4.3.

Certain pathologies result in linear abnormalities on chest X-rays. It is beyond the scope of this book to cover all these pathologies in detail. We will introduce the concept of the abnormalities and explore some of the possible causes, enabling you to "get your eye in" for these abnormalities. As with the interpretation of all abnormalities, understanding why it occurs is key to being able to confidently identify it.

TABLE 4.3. Causes of linear appearance.

Left ventricular failure	Perihilar and peripheral basal septal lines, changes acutely and resolves with diuretics
Normal ageing	Coarsening of lung markings in lower zones, no change on review of recent films
Lymphangitis	Coarse nodular and linear thickening of markings, known malignancy, often associated with pleural effusion, rapid clinical deterioration of patient
Atelectasis	Short thin lines, often basal, new on review of previous films
Subsegmental collapse	Longer thicker bands, often perihilar or basal, suggest recent infection or infarction
Scarring	Any length, persist over time unchanged
Fibrosis	Volume loss is key, persists over time

It can be very difficult to pick out a linear pattern of abnormality and it is certainly not as easy to confidently interpret as, for example, a large patch of consolidation.

Air space opacity as described in Chapter 4a is created by pathology within the alveolus or alveoli. If the abnormality is within or along the airways, with sparing of the alveolar region, then this will create linear abnormalities on the chest X-ray. Remember that there are vascular and lymphatic structures that also run within the lungs. Pathology related to these structures will therefore also appear linear. There is connective tissue between the alveoli, the airways,

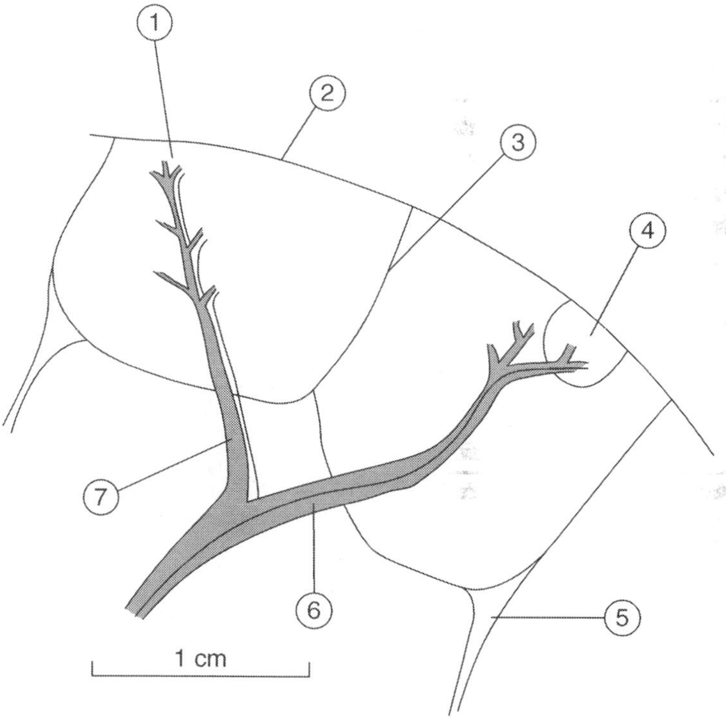

FIGURE 4.14. Diagram of secondary pulmonary lobule. (1) Terminal artery and bronchiole; (2) visceral pleura (0.1 mm); (3) interlobular septum (0.1 mm); (4) acinus (0.6–1 cm); (5) pulmonary vein (0.5 mm); (6) lobular artery (1 mm); (7) lobular bronchiole (1 mm).

the vascular structures, and the lymphatics – termed the interstitium. Abnormalities of the interstitium will also have a linear appearance. In a similar manner to the causes of air space opacity, thickening of the interstitium may result from accumulation of fluid, cellular infiltration (benign or malignant), or fibrosis.

Once again in order to understand and correctly interpret abnormalities it is important to be familiar with the basic anatomy. The secondary pulmonary lobule is the smallest lung unit marginated by connective tissue septa [1] (Fig. 4.14). While interpretation of a high-resolution CT is beyond the scope of this book, a good working knowledge of the basics is essential.

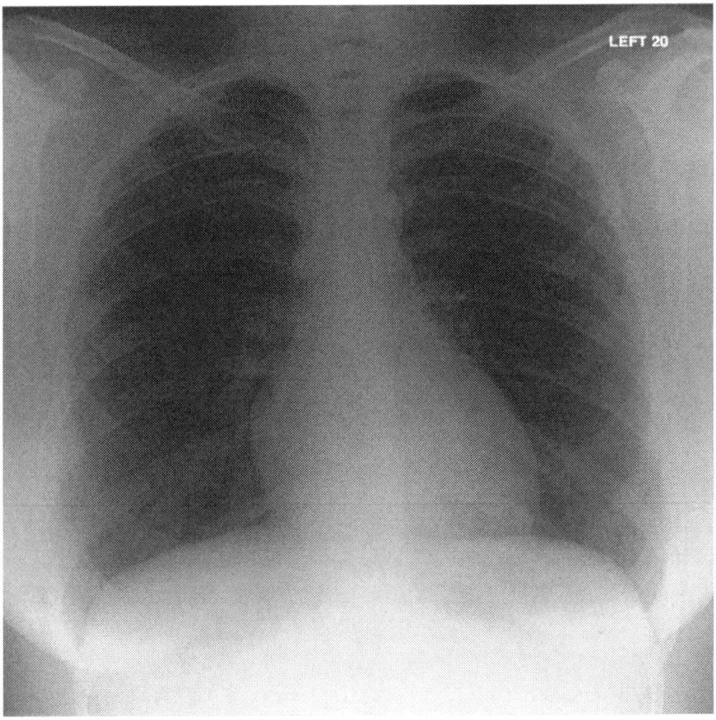

FIGURE 4.15. Normal CXR.

It is normal to see the proximal branching airways (bronchi) on a chest X-ray, but the smaller bronchioles are not seen unless caught "end on" (Fig. 4.15). They would then be seen as rings. The distal bronchioles are only seen as linear structures if abnormally thickened.

The fine branching lines seen out in the peripheral areas of a normal chest X-ray reflect vascular structures. These, however, are not seen in the most peripheral centimeter of the chest. Lines seen in the most peripheral centimeter are therefore abnormal. The interstitium is also not seen when normal and is only visualized if abnormally thickened.

4.8 Left Ventricular Failure

One of the results of left ventricular failure (LVF) is the accumulation of fluid in the interstitium along the lines of the airways. This abnormal thickening is demonstrated as lines within the perihilar region. These lines are termed "septal lines." If they occur in a central and perihilar distribution, they are termed "deep septal lines." These correspond to the lines described by Kerley as A lines. Septal lines occurring in the periphery, often at the costophrenic angles, are the so-called Kerley B lines (Fig. 4.16a).

Peripheral septal lines are usually horizontal and typically about 1 cm long. If they have a rapid onset of appearance they are almost diagnostic of pulmonary oedema. If they appear gradually over a period of time, other causes of interstitial thickening will need to be considered, for example, fibrosis or lymphangitis carcinomatosis.

As the extent of the oedema progresses, fluid will start to accumulate in the air spaces. This initially gives a ground glass appearance and eventually air space opacity and consolidation as previously described (Fig. 4.16b).

a

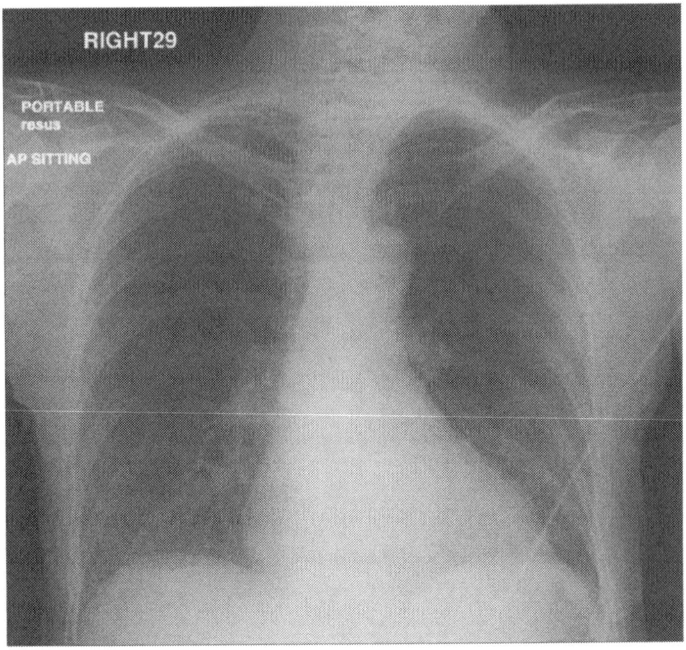

FIGURE 4.16a. Left ventricular failure. Note perihilar and basal linear opacities (Kerly A and B).

b

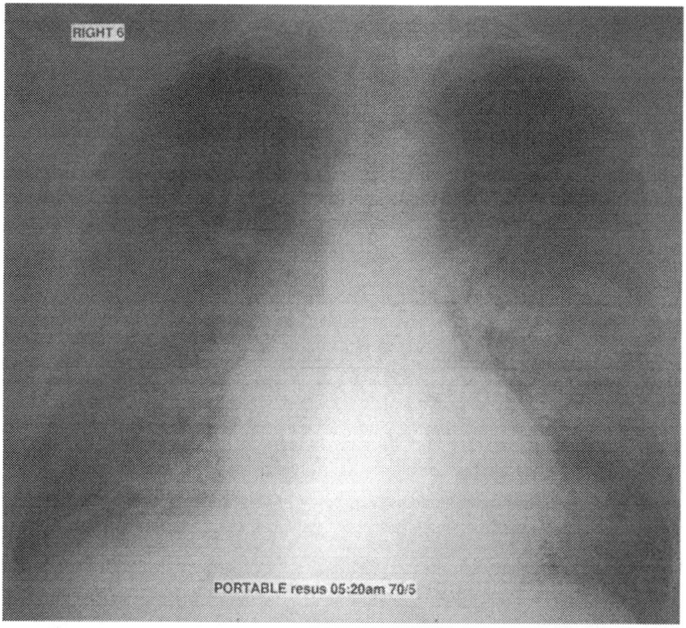

FIGURE 4.16b. Left ventricular failure. Note perihilar and basal ground glass opacity and perihilar septal lines (Kerly A) and basal lines (Kerly B).

Fluid may be seen in the horizontal fissure of the right lung, thickening its appearance, and pleural effusions are commonly also seen.

4.9 Normal Ageing Lungs

With ageing there are some predictable changes in the appearances of the lungs. It is normal for the lung markings to become reduced within the upper zones and a generalized coarsening to occur within the lower zones. It is important that this is not overinterpreted as either upper zone emphysema or evidence of a lower zone reticulation created by fibrosis. If there is doubt comparison can be made with previous films and correlation made with the clinical findings (Fig. 4.17).

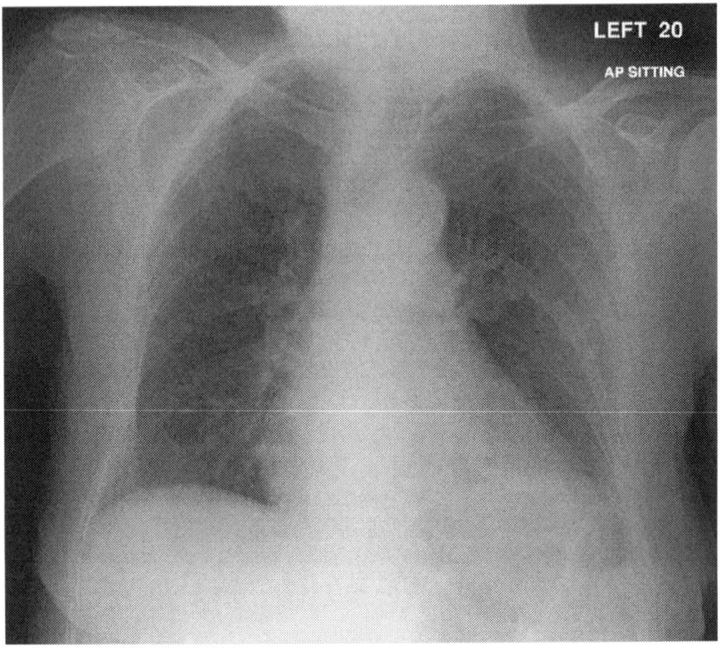

FIGURE 4.17. Normal ageing lungs.

4.10 Lymphangitis Carcinomatosis

Lymphangitis carcinomatosis is not a common condition, but it is important to be aware of its appearances and at least consider the diagnosis in the context of a known malignancy. It occurs most commonly in breast and lung cancers. Patients often present with a sub-acute deterioration. The radiological abnormalities include a coarse reticulation with often a slightly nodular appearance, which may be demonstrated to have worsened on a series of chest X-rays. There may be accompanying pleural effusions, unilateral or bilateral (Fig. 4.18).

There are typical appearances on high-resolution CT. As the disease process involves the lymphatics there is an abnormality that traces the course of the lymphatic system.

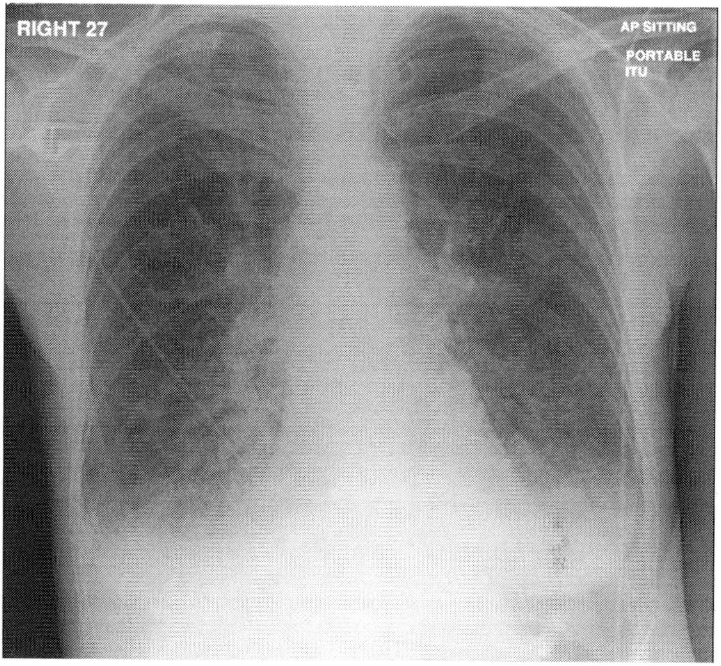

FIGURE 4.18. Lymphangitis carcinomatosis.

4.11 Fibrosis

There are many conditions that lead to pulmonary fibrosis Table 4.4, although it may be idiopathic. This book will not attempt to cover the causes in detail, but will give an approach to identification of the radiological abnormality, allowing diagnosis.

The pathological process of fibrosis involves a thickening of the interstitium of the lung. It is not normally possible to see the interstitium on a plain chest X-ray as these structures are too small and beyond the limit of resolution. Thickening of the interstitium, as caused by fibrosis, results in it becoming visible and this is demonstrated as lines which may be quite subtle and are often irregular. Conglomeration can lead to a nodular appearance. The combination of overlying lines is termed reticulation. The superimposition of nodules will result in a reticular nodular abnormality.

The pathological process of fibrosis results in a "stiffening up" of the lungs which cannot inflate normally and therefore volume loss occurs. Comparison can be made with previous imaging, but it is important to ensure that the patient has taken an adequate breath in. Pulmonary fibrosis can be difficult to differentiate radiologically from left ventricular failure (as can be the case clinically). It may be necessary to make a correlation with the clinical findings and a history of breathlessness and inspiratory crackles are useful indicators. In addition there is often a long history of progressive disease in pulmonary fibrosis with a frequently shorter disease span in left ventricular failure.

The key abnormalities in pulmonary fibrosis are the presence of reticulation and volume loss. Comparison with serial films can be very helpful. If plain film findings are suggestive of pulmonary fibrosis and the clinical picture and lung function tests are concordant, then further examination with HRCT should be performed.

Particular causes of fibrosis result in different geographical locations of disease predominance. Some affect the mid zones more than the lower zones and vice versa.

The classification of pulmonary fibrosis is relatively complex and there is some discordance between the terms used by various groups of doctors.

4.12 Lower Zone Fibrosis

The chest X-ray shows a predominantly lower zone abnormality, in keeping with a basal distribution of fibrosis. The differential diagnosis for these appearances would include cryptogenic fibrosing alveolitis, fibrosis related to connective tissue diseases, drug-induced fibrosis, asbestos-related fibrosis, and any cause of so-called usual interstitial pneumonitis (UIP) (Fig. 4.19).

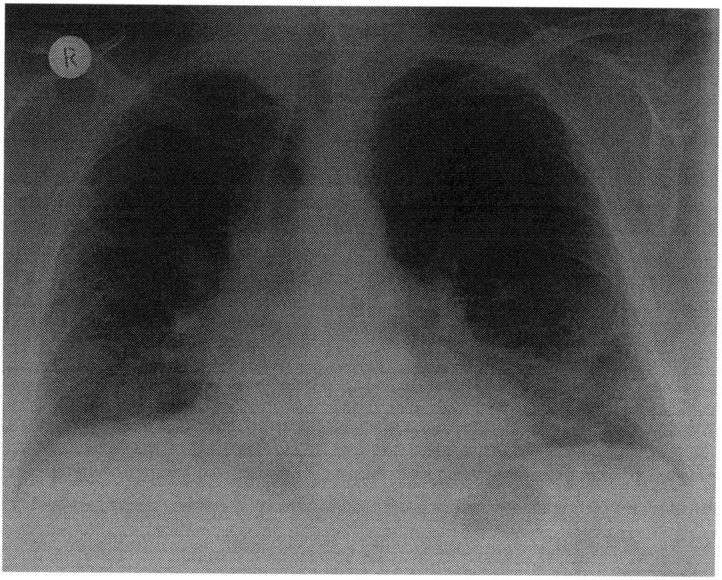

FIGURE 4.19. Lower zone fibrosis.

4.13 Upper Zone Fibrosis

The X-ray demonstrates loss of volume within the upper zones as evidenced by superior displacement of the hilar regions bilaterally. There is an upper zone reticulation (Fig. 4.20).

There is relative sparing of the lower zones and tenting of the hemi-diaphragms as a result of the upper lobe volume loss.

There is a differential diagnosis for the causes of these appearances; in this case the disease process is chronic extrinsic allergic alveolitis (cEAA). Other causes of predominantly upper zone fibrosis include previous tuberculosis, ankylosing spondylitis, fibrosis related to pneumoconiosis, and previous radiotherapy.

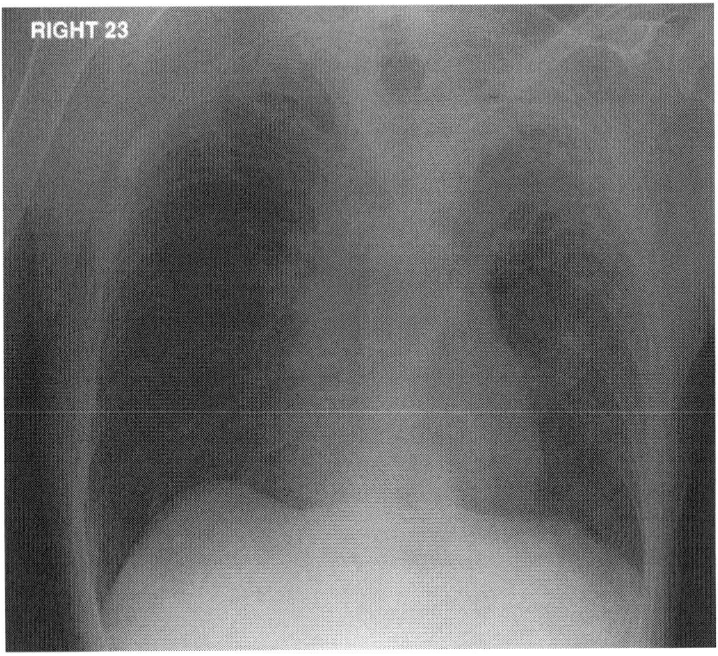

FIGURE 4.20. Upper zone fibrosis.

4.14 Mid Zone Fibrosis

Note the very coarse linear abnormality in a predominant perihilar distribution. There may be multiple nodules and confluent opacities present (Fig. 4.21).

The typical cause for mid zone fibrosis is sarcoidosis and with progression of time the disease process does begin to involve the upper and lower zones.

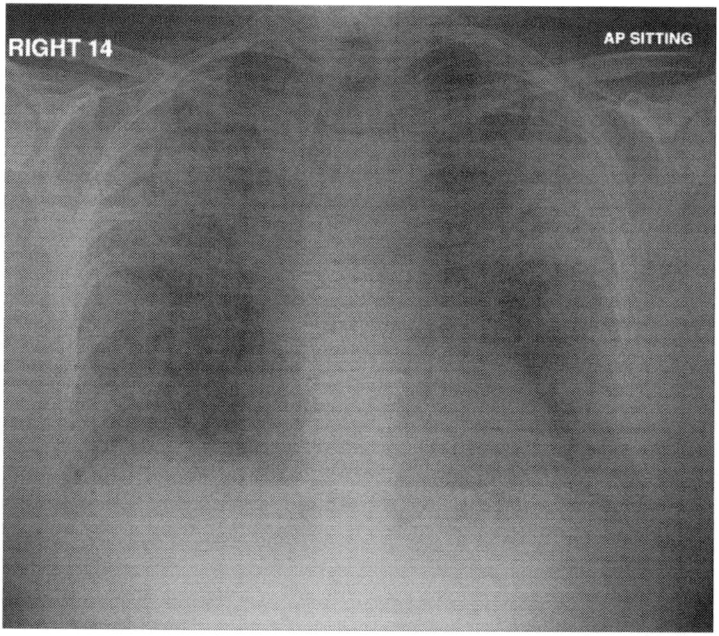

FIGURE 4.21. Mid zone fibrosis.

TABLE 4.4. Causes of fibrosis.

Upper zone fibrosis	Lower zone fibrosis	Mid zone fibrosis
Tuberculosis	Usual interstitial pneumonitis	Sarcoidosis
Chronic extrinsic allergic alveolitis	Asbestos-related fibrosis	
Radiotherapy	Drug-induced fibrosis (most commonly)	
Ankylosing spondylitis		
Progressive massive fibrosis		
Histoplasmosis		

Some lines on chest X-rays do not conform to the above patterns and these may be evidence of scarring due to previous lung insult or more focal areas of lung collapse.

4.15 Subsegmental Collapse

Collapse of the lung may be limited to a small part of a segment of a lobe, termed subsegmental. This results in a focal region of discrete long lines. In the acute setting this can be related to infection or infarction and comparison with old films may be useful. Once the acute abnormality resolves there is often persistence of the linear abnormality, suggesting the presence of established infarction or scarring (Fig. 4.22).

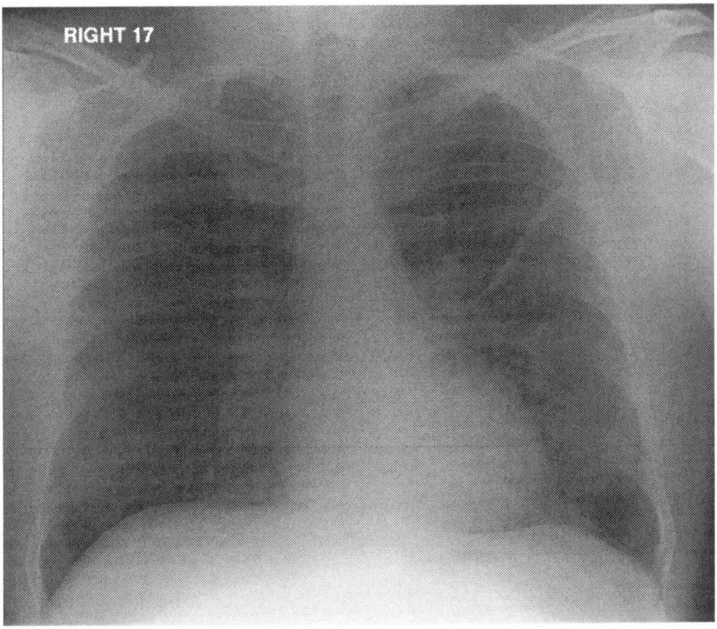

FIGURE 4.22. Subsegmental collapse.

4.16 Scarring

Scars may simply appear as thin lines, a clue to their nature is persistence with time (Fig. 4.23).

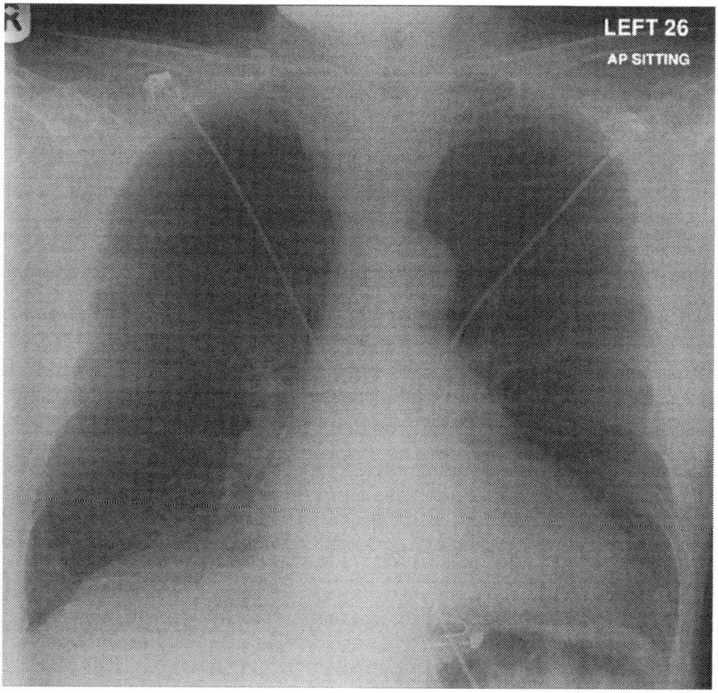

FIGURE 4.23. Right basal scarring.

4.17 Atelectasis

Basal atelectasis is due to collapse of small peripheral airways and alveoli. It may be a temporary phenomenon and will resolve if, for example, it is due to an infection with a degree of mucus plugging. On the chest X-ray it appears as short thin lines and is often basal, although it can occur anywhere within the lung. If it is a new phenomenon, then it is usually suggestive of a recent infection. Resolution often occurs on follow-up (Figs. 4.24a and b).

a

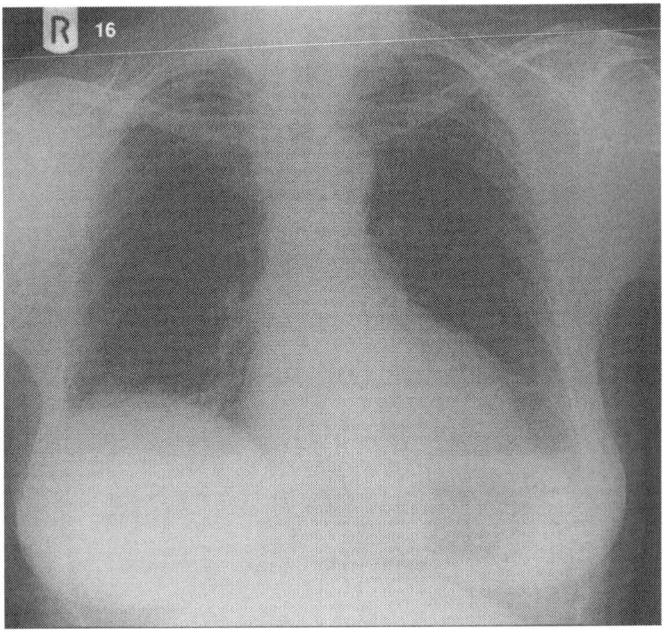

FIGURE 4.24. (continued).

b

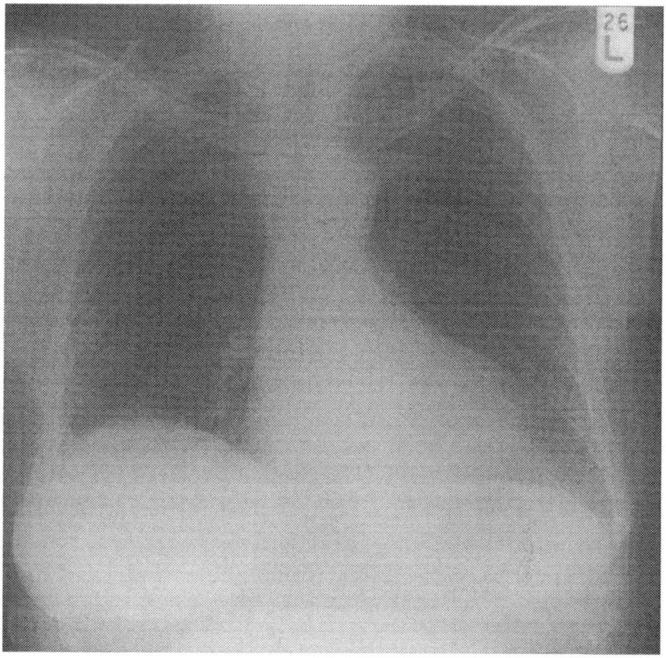

FIGURE 4.24. (a) Basal atelectasis (b) following resolution.

4.18 Key Points

1) Linear (reticular) abnormality is due to pathology involving airways, lymphatics, veins, and the interstitium of the lung.
2) Comparison with previous films is helpful to determine the cause.
3) Different pathologies result in particular patterns of linear abnormality.
4) Volume loss is a key finding in fibrosis.

Reference

1. Miller WS. *The Lung*. Springfield, IL: Charles C Thomas Publisher, 1947:39–42.

Chapter 4d
Nodules

Many disease processes result in the appearance of nodules on a chest X-ray. It is not always possible to determine the exact cause from a single plain film. Recognition of a pattern of abnormality will, however, enable a reasonable differential of the appearances to be drawn up.

Nodules may not always be easy to see. A large dense opacity in the middle of a lung is likely to be recognized. Nodules, however, can be very subtle and can be single or multiple. Spotting the presence of nodules can make a significant difference if they are recognized in a timely fashion.

As with many things, it is experience that enables the observer to pick up subtle changes on a chest X-ray. Some nodules do fall into the group of abnormalities that are difficult to see and therefore are easy to miss. Having a structured approach to chest X-ray interpretation, you are more likely to be able to spot abnormalities. This should lead to increased confidence and in time, greater experience. Remember that even nodules which are easy to see require sensible interpretation.

If it is suspected that a nodule or nodules are present on a film, but a degree of uncertainty remains, the following method of analysis may help:

I) Compare the current film with old films – has there been a change in the appearance and over what time interval.
II) Assess the area of lung demarcated between the anterior and posterior ribs, as this helps eliminate bone.
III) Apical views may help in the demonstration of apical nodules.

IV) If doubt persists discuss the film with a radiologist in terms of possible further investigations.

The chest X-ray examples that we give are grouped according to solitary or multiple nodules. This gives a general, but not exhaustive, overview.

4.19 Solitary Pulmonary Nodule

There are several factors to consider when assessing a solitary pulmonary nodule:

1. Is it smooth? This generally favours a benign cause, but it is not a fail safe. A spiculated appearance is highly suspicious for carcinoma.
2. Is there associated calcification? This favours a benign cause.
3. Was it present on previous films, and if so has it changed? If unchanged over a period of months or years, it is unlikely to be of any significance. If it is a new feature in comparison to old films, this raises your index of suspicion.
4. Location, location, location. Hilar and upper lobe nodules have a higher index of suspicion for malignancy.
5. Size does matter. The larger the nodule, the more the suspicion for malignancy.
6. Are there any other associated abnormalities on the film? Lymph node enlargement within the mediastinum or rib destruction/erosion all favour malignancy.
7. Is there any evidence of cavitation? This is particularly common in squamous cell carcinoma and secondaries, although nodules from benign causes such as rheumatoid arthritis, Wegener's granulomatosis, and infarction can cavitate (Table 4.5).

There is published evidence-based guidance for follow-up of a solitary pulmonary nodule (Table 4.6).

TABLE 4.5. Appearance of nodules suggesting benign and malignant features.

Benign	Malignant
Smooth outline	Irregular/spiculate outline
Presence of calcification	Uncalcified
Lower zone	Hilar or upper zone location
Small, no increase over time	Large, > 1 cm or increasing in size
No cavitation	Cavitation
No other features of malignancy	Ancillary features, e.g., bone erosion

TABLE 4.6. Fleischner Society pulmonary nodules recommendations.

Nodule size (mm)	Low-risk patients	High-risk patients
≤4	No follow-up needed	Follow-up at 12 months. If no change, no further imaging needed
>4–6	Follow-up at 12 months. If no change, no further imaging needed	Initial follow-up CT at 6–12 months and then at 18–24 months if no change
>6–8	Initial follow-up CT at 6–12 months and then at 18–24 months if no change	Initial follow-up CT at 3–6 months and then at 9–12 and 24 months if no change
>8	Follow-up CT at around 3, 9, and 24 months. Dynamic contrast-enhanced CT, PET, and/or biopsy	Same as for low-risk patients

Low-risk patients: Minimal or absent history of smoking and other known risk factors.
High-risk patients: History of smoking or other known risk factors.
Adapted from Heber MacMahon et al., Radiology 2005 237:395–400

4.19.1 Benign Nodules

4.19.1.1 Hamartoma

Note the typical "popcorn" calcification. This nodule remained unchanged over a period of several chest X-rays. It is a benign nodule of no clinical significance (Fig. 4.25).

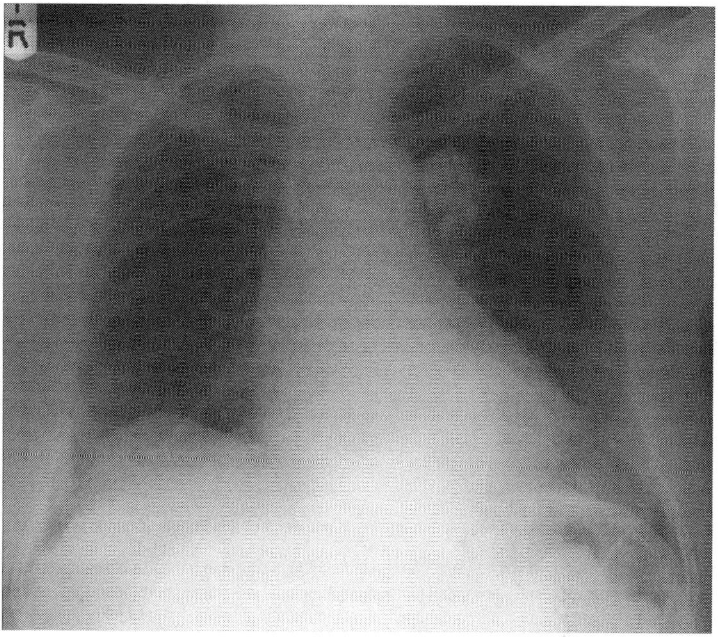

FIGURE 4.25. Hamartoma.

4.19.1.2 Wegener's Granulomatosis

The nodules in a Wegener's granulomatosis may be single or multiple and can cavitate. Correlation with the clinical history will help in identification, but the nodules themselves are not specifically of a different appearance to other cavitatory nodules (Fig. 4.26).

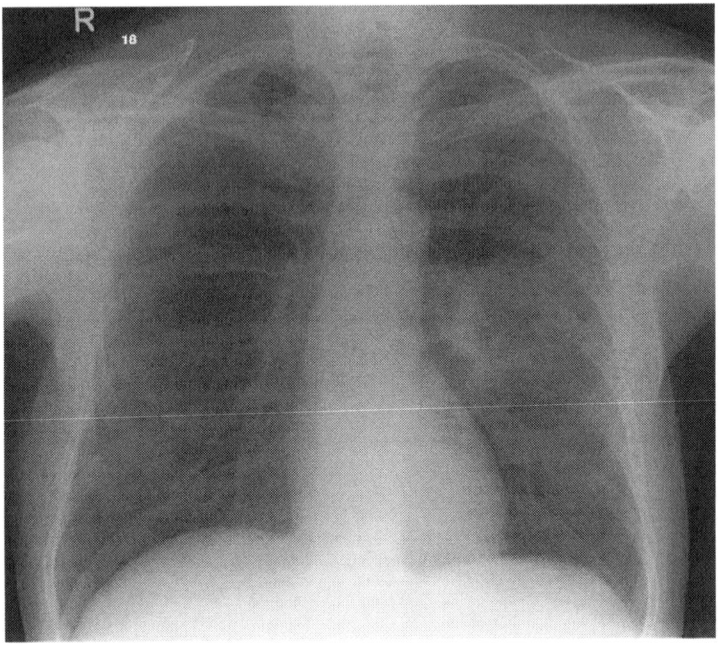

FIGURE 4.26. Wegener's nodule.

4.19.1.3 Abscess

Abscesses can often be well defined on chest X-rays as they have relatively thick walls. Note the presence of an air fluid level. The abscess itself may be a result of a malignant process and so it is important to ensure that follow-up occurs (Fig. 4.27).

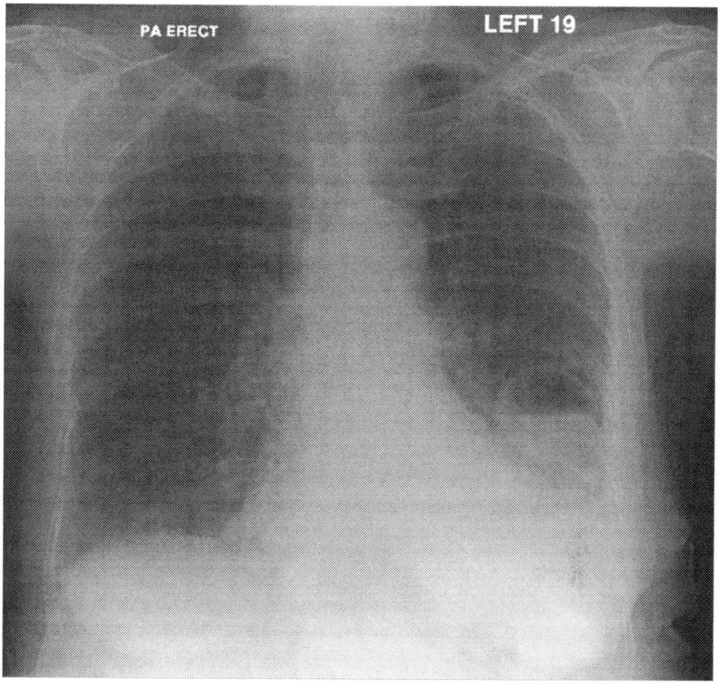

FIGURE 4.27. Lung abscess with left basal consolidation.

4.19.2 Malignant Nodules

Note the dense irregular mass at the hilum. Patients may have typical presenting symptoms of haemoptysis and/or weight loss, but may just have a cough. The overwhelming majority of patients are smokers (Fig. 4.28).

There is a left apical primary bronchogenic carcinoma with destruction of the fourth left posterior rib (Fig. 4.29). The adjacent rib destruction gives a very high index of suspicion for malignancy. Benign processes may cause pressure erosion, but frank destruction reflects malignancy. It is easy to miss the bony involvement unless you always look for it.

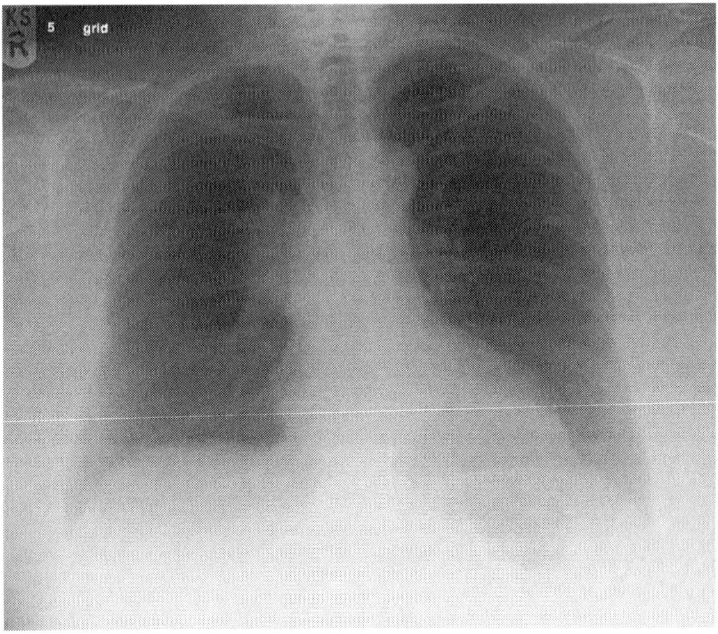

FIGURE 4.28. Right hilar bronchogenic carcinoma.

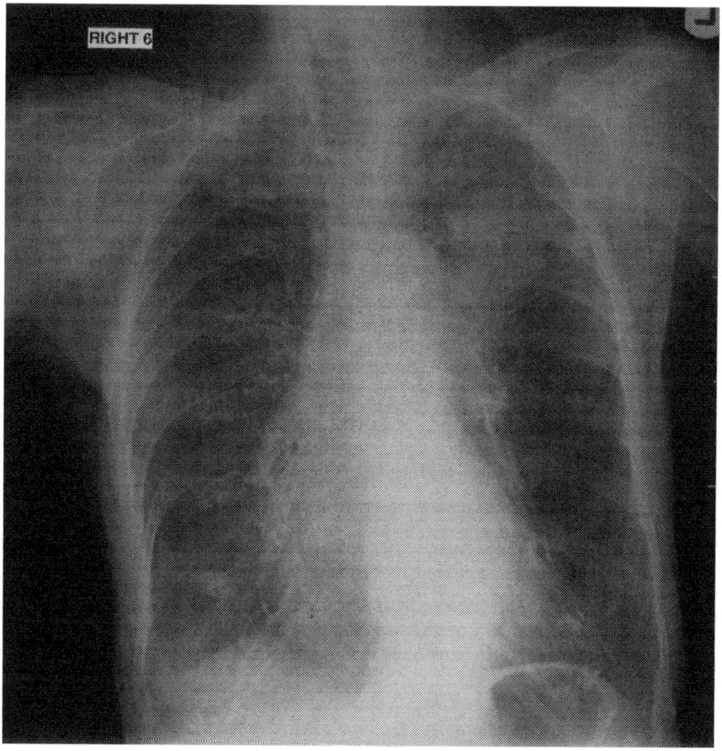

FIGURE 4.29. Left apical mass with destruction of the fourth left posterior rib.

4.20 Multiple Pulmonary Nodules

4.20.1 Benign Nodules

4.20.1.1 Miliary Tuberculosis

Note that the nodules are tiny, ≤2 mm. There is an even distribution throughout both lungs (Fig. 4.30).

Other diseases that can cause a "miliary" appearance include histoplasmosis, haemosiderosis, and multiple metastases, particularly from thyroid carcinoma.

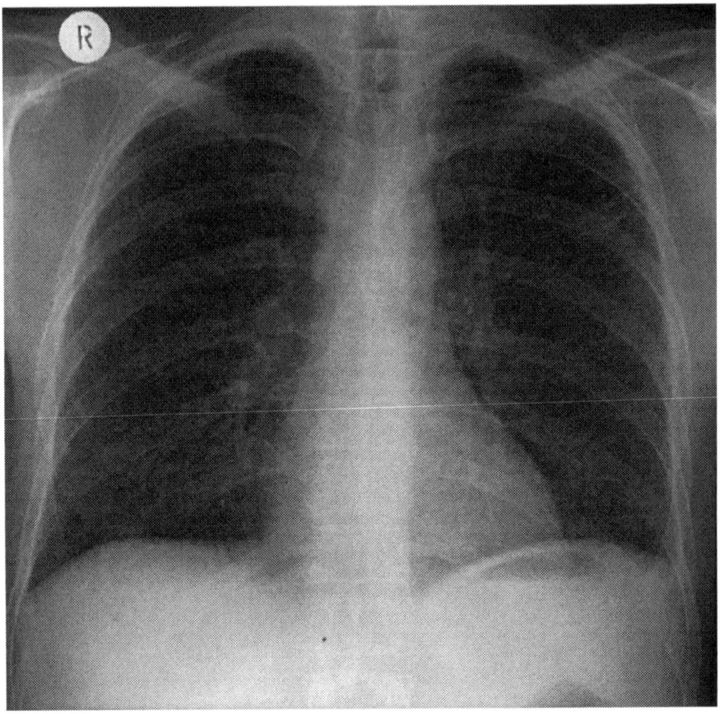

FIGURE 4.30. Miliary TB.

4.20.1.2 Sarcoidosis

The nodularity is often subtle and the patient, although breathless, is otherwise generally well. The abnormality usually occurs with a perihilar distribution. There may be associated enlargement of the hilar nodes, and while diagnostically classical this is not essential (Fig. 4.31).

The radiological diagnosis of sarcoidosis is best made using HRCT.

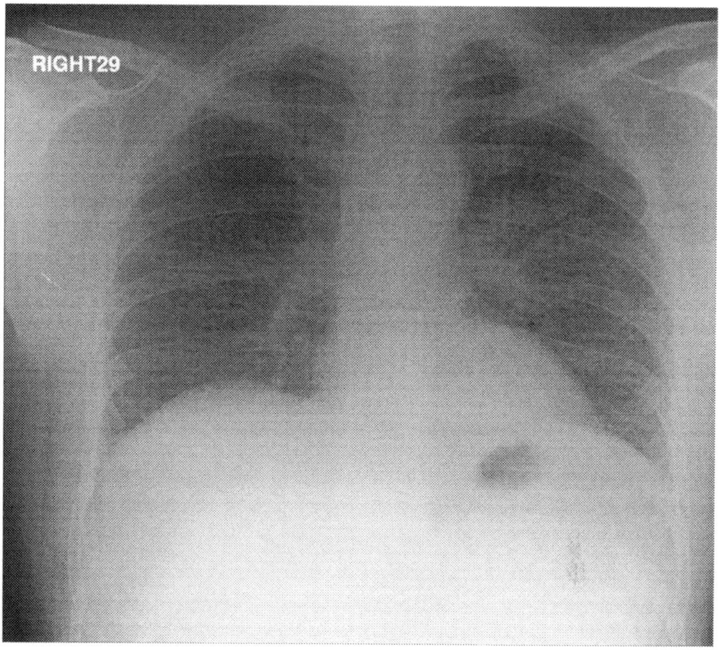

FIGURE 4.31. Sarcoidosis.

4.20.1.3 Infection

There may be branching nodularity suggestive of infection which can be associated with bronchiectasis. Infection in particular areas such as the apical segments of upper or lower lobes raises the suspicion of tuberculosis (Fig. 4.32a). A branching nodularity may also be caused by mucus plugging.

Multiple calcified nodules can be a late appearance of previous chicken pox infection (Fig. 4.32b) or TB (granulomata).

a

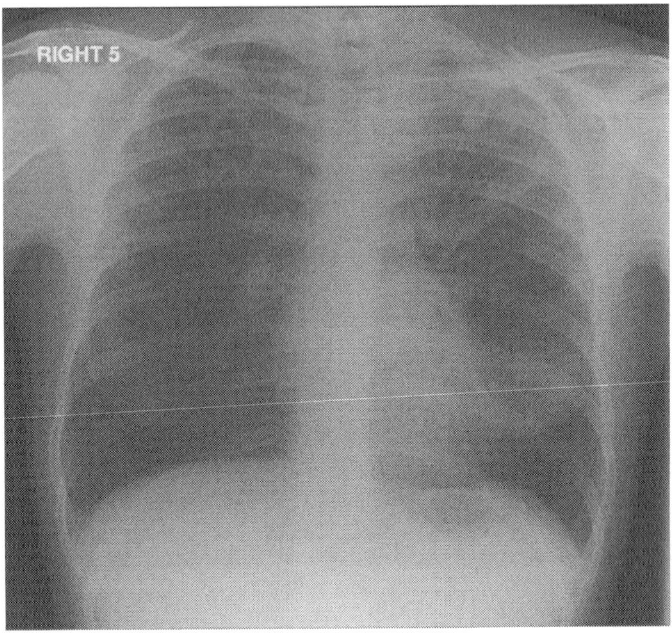

FIGURE 4.32. (continued).

b

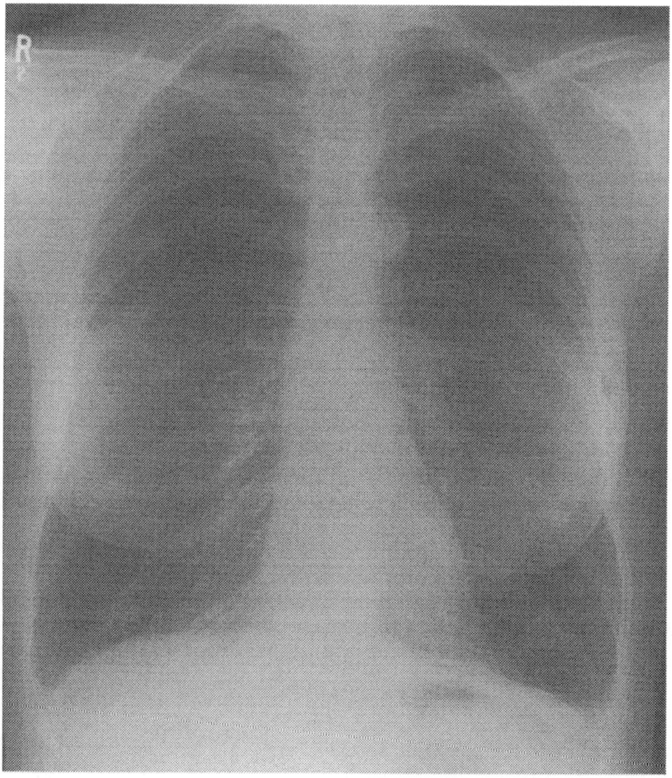

FIGURE 4.32. Infection. (a) Active TB. Note bilateral apical nodules with right-sided cavity; (b) calcified nodules post-chicken pox.

4.20.2 Malignant

Note the random distribution and variation in size (Fig. 4.33a). Extension of the nodularity to the pleural surface is an indicator of malignancy and most benign causes of nodules do not extend this far although it may be seen in subpleural sarcoid. Some metastases have particular patterns, for example, renal cell carcinoma has a very round appearance, termed "cannonball metastases," (Fig. 4.33b) and squamous cell metastases often cavitate.

The recognition and correct interpretation of a nodule or nodules help to ensure that appropriate further investigations are performed within a suitable time frame.

Most nodules, if new or enlarging or of a significant size on first presentation, will need to be further assessed with CT and may require biopsy.

a

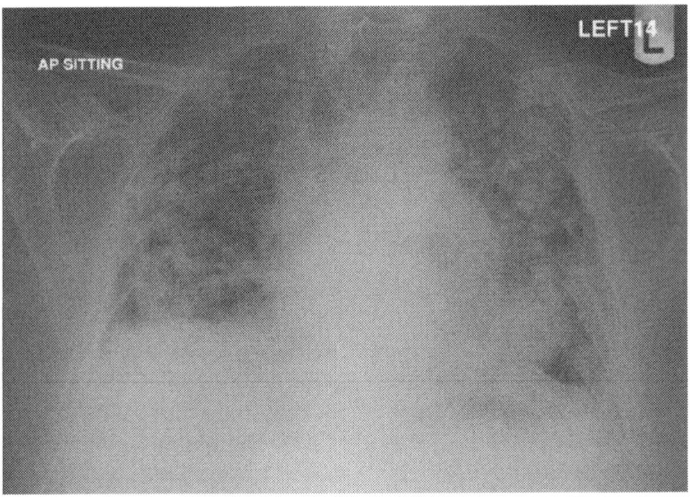

FIGURE 4.33. (continued).

b

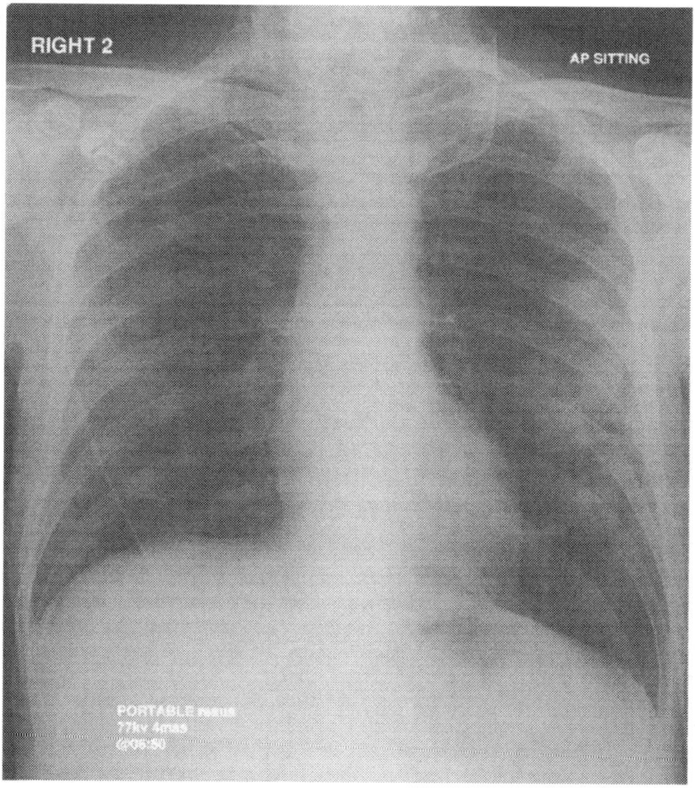

FIGURE 4.33. (a) Multiple small metastases of varying size; (b) "cannonball" metastases.

4.21 Key Points

1) Nodules may be subtle, check review areas.
2) Certain features suggest a benign or malignant cause, however, are not specific and further investigation, e.g., biopsy, may be required.
3) Comparison with old films is key.
4) Location, distribution, and size are important features.
5) Look for secondary features of malignancy.

Chapter 4e
Rings and Holes

There are several abnormalities which result in a chest X-ray appearance of either rings or holes. While the underlying pathologies are diverse, the approach to assessment of the abnormalities on the chest X-ray is similar. In all cases, what is demonstrated on the chest X-ray is a reduction in lung markings giving the configuration of a ring or a hole, depending on its cause. It is worth noting that a reduction in lung markings may simply be a reflection of the normal ageing process, particularly in the upper zones.

It is in general more difficult to appreciate an abnormality as the absence of something, as opposed to the presence of something. It is therefore a matter of training the eye to appreciate a reduction in the normal lung markings and this will allow you to identify a well-defined cyst, the "ring" of a dilated airway, or the presence of a large bulla.

What follows is not an exhaustive list, but includes examples of the more common abnormalities.

In this example there is hyperinflation of the lungs, a general reduction of lung markings within the upper zones, and crowding of lung markings in the lower zones (Fig. 4.34).

In this example there are well-defined bullae at the apices. These are thin walled areas of destroyed lung. As in this case, they are usually within the upper zones but once extensive can extend into the lower zones. Crowding of lung markings occurs around bullae as they take up physical space (Fig. 4.35).

Alpha-1-antitrypsin deficiency is a hereditary condition which results in emphysema that affects predominantly the lower zones. It often occurs in non-smokers. In this example

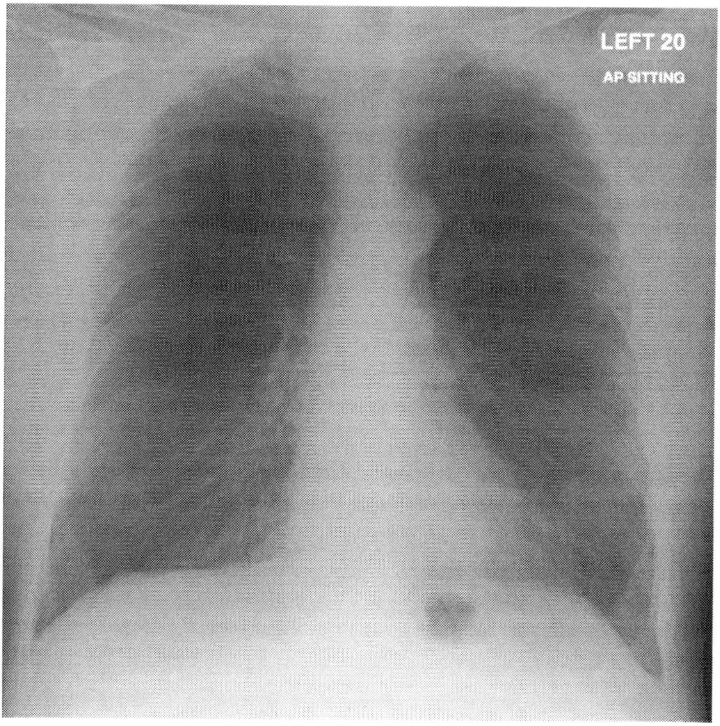

FIGURE 4.34. Upper lobe emphysema.

there are established lower zone bullae with crowding of adjacent lung markings (Fig. 4.36).

Bronchiectasis is the dilatation of airways which can be a late consequence of childhood infection. Often there is no obvious cause. The dilated airways are best seen with high-resolution CT scanning but can sometimes be seen on a CXR as rings (Fig. 4.37). These rings are end-on dilated airways. They may or may not be thick walled, depending on the presence or absence of mucosal thickening. "Tram lines" are dilated airways seen along their length usually in the lower zones.

In this example ring opacities are noted in the upper lobes. Basal nodules are also present due to current infection (Fig. 4.38).

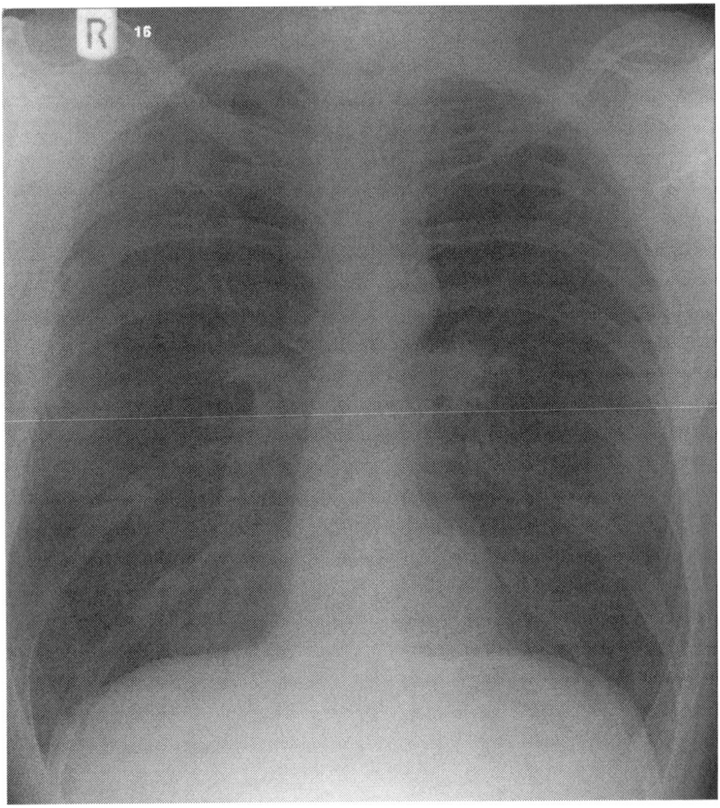

FIGURE 4.35. Emphysema with apical bullae.

A thin-walled cavity (as opposed to cavitating mass) is present within the right upper lobe. It contains a soft tissue ball which is an aspergilloma. This is often better demonstrated with CT where the aspergilloma is seen to move between supine and prone scans. Note the background of fibrosis (Fig. 4.39).

More unusual causes of cystic abnormalities are beyond the scope of this book. These would include conditions such as lymphocytic interstitial pneumonitis (LIP) often related to connective tissue disorders (Fig. 4.40) and lymphangiomyomatosis (LAM). These latter conditions are typically investigated with HRCT.

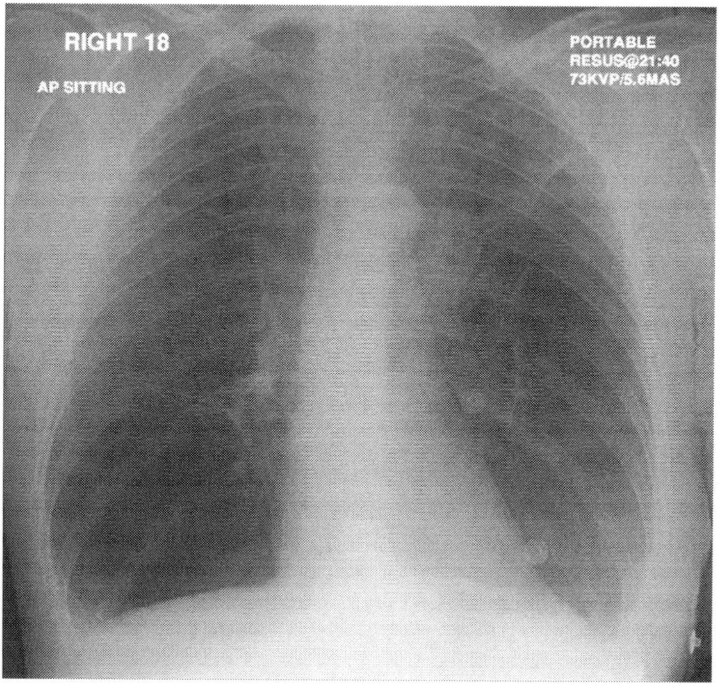

FIGURE 4.36. Alpha-1-antitrypsin deficiency with basal emphysema.

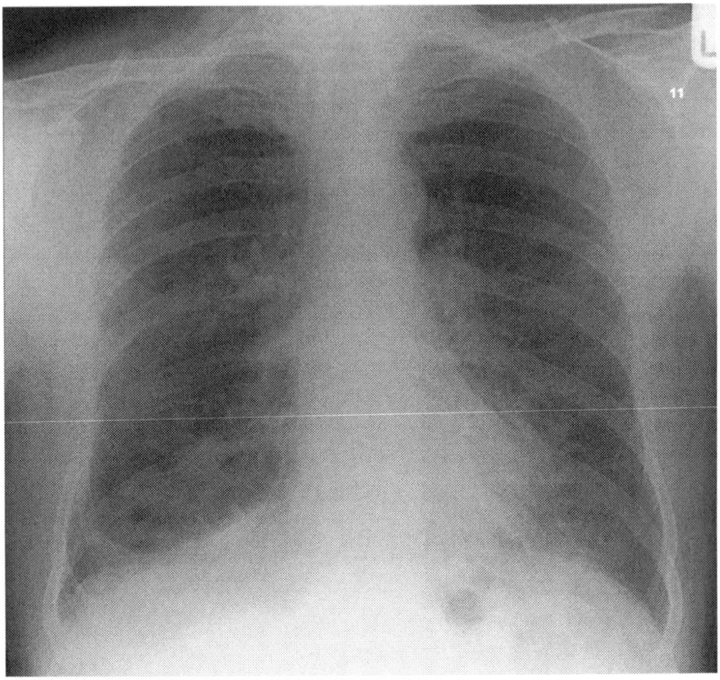

FIGURE 4.37. Bronchiectasis, note the ring opacities particularly within right lower zone.

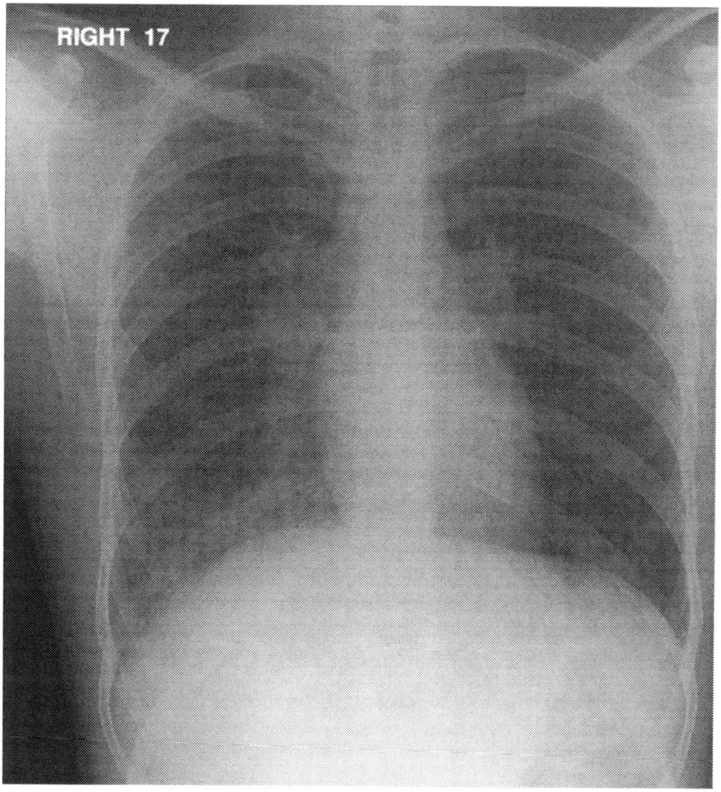

FIGURE 4.38. Cystic fibrosis with ring opacities within the upper zones due to bronchiectasis and nodules at the right lung base due to current infection. The lungs are hyperinflated.

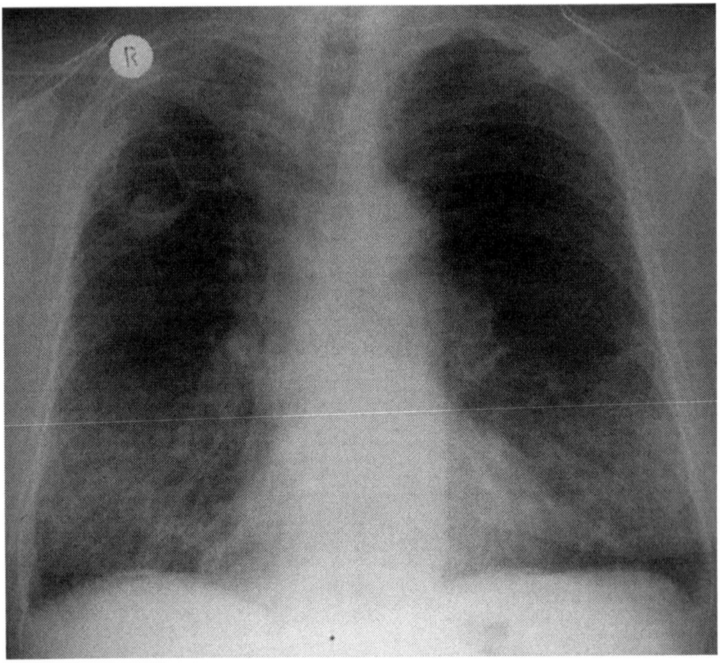

FIGURE 4.39. Right apical aspergilloma with a background of pulmonary fibrosis.

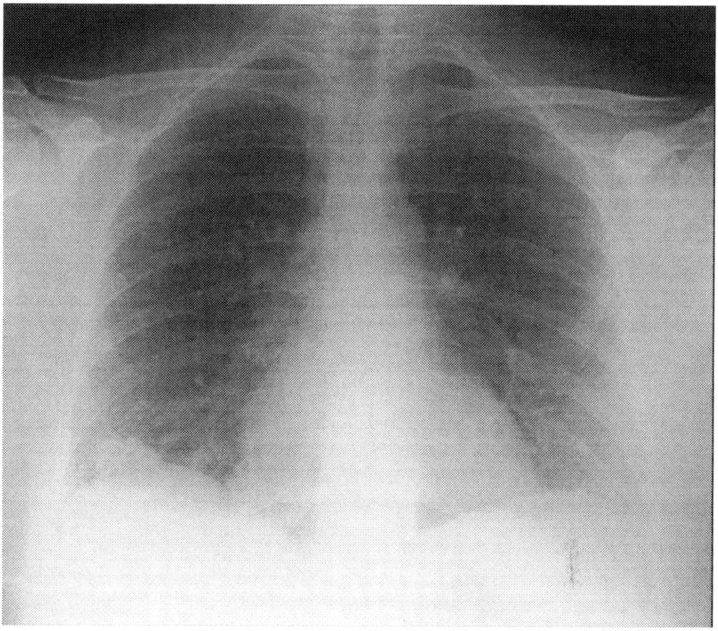

FIGURE 4.40. Thin-walled cyst in a patient with scleroderma and LIP, note thin-walled cyst below left hilum and right basal parenchymal calcification which is another feature of scleroderma.

4.22 Key Points

1) The abnormality may be a relative reduction in normal lung markings.
2) Cysts and emphysematous bullae are thin walled.
3) If emphysema is predominantly basal consider alpha-1-antitrypsin deficiency.

Chapter 5
The Pleura

Pleural Abnormalities

Pleural abnormalities are a common finding on chest X-ray, the significance of which varies from trivial to marked. In order to ensure that such abnormalities are not missed, it is important that all check areas are examined on each chest X-ray. Some abnormalities of the pleura can be subtle and may be missed. Typical areas to identify pleural abnormalities are at the costophrenic and cardiophrenic angles, the apices, and the peripheral outline of both lungs.

Three main categories of pleural abnormalities are seen: effusions, pleural thickening or calcification, and pneumothoraces. These are dealt with separately in the following sections, and in the first section we will consider pleural effusions.

R. Joarder, N. Crundwell (eds.), *Chest X-Ray in Clinical Practice*,
DOI 10.1007/978-1-84882-099-9_5,

Chapter 5a
Pleural Effusions

Pleural effusions are a common finding. Further investigation of a pleural effusion, in addition to a detailed history and examination, may include a pleural tap. This establishes whether the effusion is a result of an exudate or a transudate. This knowledge further helps elucidate the cause of the effusion Table 5.1.

We will be limiting our discussion to the chest X-ray findings, although clearly interpretation needs to be made within the clinical context of the patient.

The typical findings of an effusion are opacity at the lung base with a meniscal appearance laterally at the costophrenic angle. If the effusion is small, it may be difficult to be certain that the abnormality is not simply related to minor thickening of the pleura. Comparison with previous films can be very useful. If the abnormality is longstanding and unchanged, thickening is more likely. If doubt persists, examination with ultrasound is a very sensitive method of demonstrating fluid.

A moderate effusion is usually easier to identify as a fluid level, with again a laterally placed meniscus (Fig. 5.1). It is also usually accompanied by significant signs and symptoms.

A very large effusion may cause complete opacification of the affected hemi-thorax. This can be differentiated from complete collapse of the lung (see Fig. 4.13) as the mediastinum will not move toward the affected side, indeed the mass effect of the effusion may have displaced the mediastinum away from it (Fig. 5.2).

The causes of pleural effusions are multiple and we have grouped them broadly into benign and malignant.

TABLE 5.1. Common causes of pleural effusions.

Transudate (often bilateral, pleura normal)	Exudate (often unilateral, pleura abnormal)
LVF	Infection
Fluid overload	Infarction
Hypoalbuminemia, e.g., cirrhosis, nephrotic syndrome	Malignancy
	Inflammation, e.g., Rheumatoid arthritis, systemic lupus erythematosus
	Ascites, e.g., cirrhosis, Meigs syndrome
	Traumatic, e.g., chest trauma, oesophageal rupture
	Rare causes, e.g., yellow nail syndrome

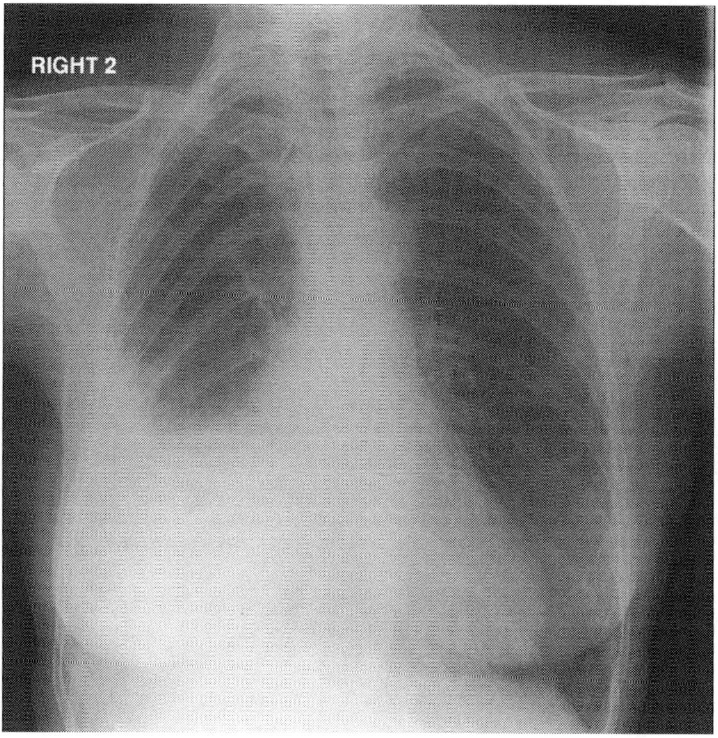

FIGURE 5.1. Moderate right pleural effusion. Note the blunting of the costophrenic angle, a laterally placed meniscus, and loss of clarity of the lung and outline of the hemi-diaphragm.

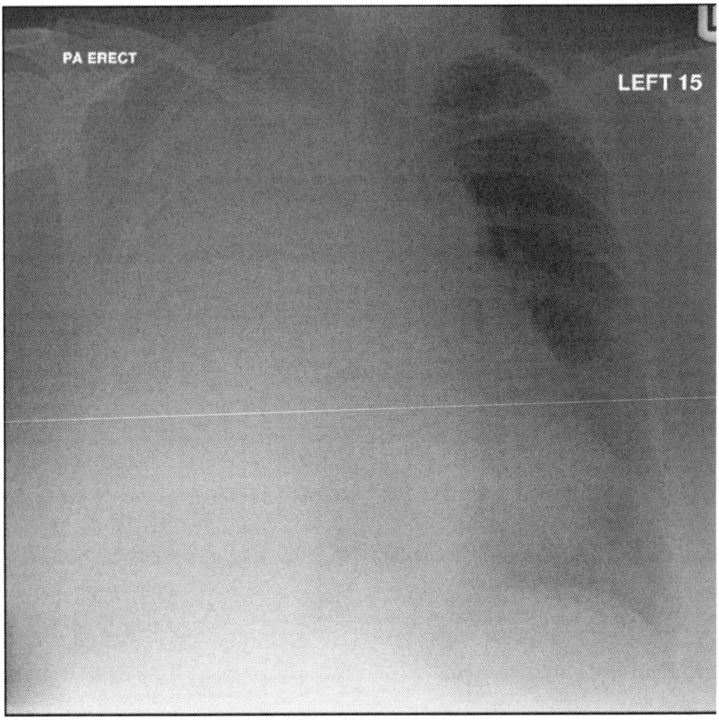

FIGURE 5.2. Large right pleural effusion. Note the mediastinal shift away from the effusion.

5.1 Benign Pleural Effusion

This is usually classified into a unilateral or bilateral effusion.

5.1.1 Unilateral

A unilateral pleural effusion is generally more significant than bilateral and will require further investigation to exclude a malignant cause.

Common benign causes include infection and infarction. It may be impossible to elucidate a cause from the chest X-ray

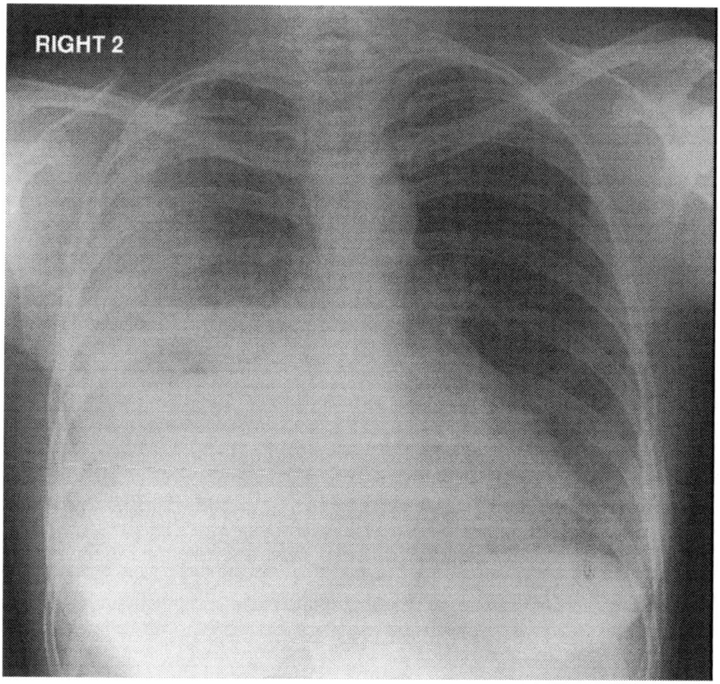

FIGURE 5.3. Right pleural effusion with mid zone consolidation.

alone and clinical history and examination play their part. Radiological clues to infection include consolidation which may be visible at the superior aspect of an effusion or elsewhere on the chest X-ray (Fig. 5.3). Infarction may also be associated with consolidation, classically wedge shaped. This is, however, rarely present and often the chest X-ray is normal in a case of pulmonary embolism. Infarction typically gives a blood-stained tap.

Traumatic effusions are also likely to contain blood and there is usually an appropriate clinical context. There may be adjacent rib fractures or hydro-pneumothorax. Empyemas may resemble simple pleural effusions, but are often loculated and tethered (Fig. 5.4). Occasionally these extend upward toward the apex, without occupying the whole pleural space and giving a large, but peripheral, appearance. They may be associated with a rind of pleural thickening, which

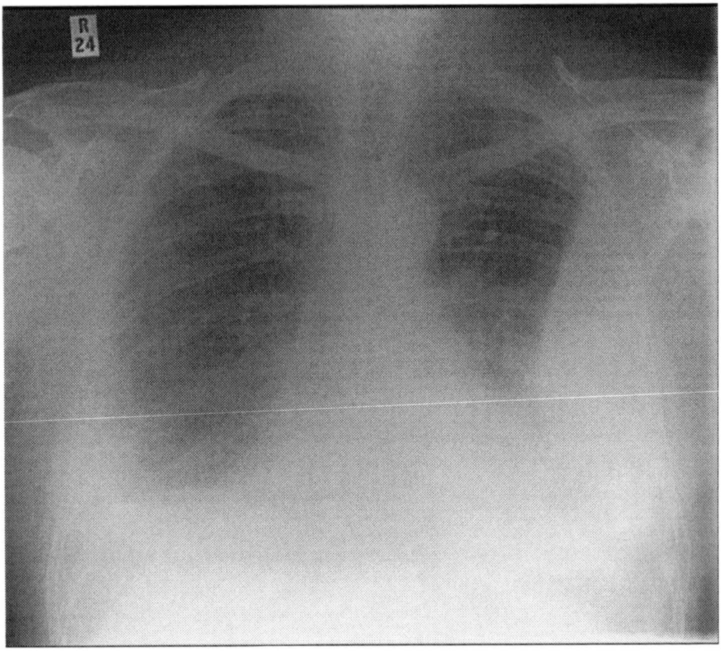

FIGURE 5.4. Empyema. There is dense pleural opacification. This continues up the lateral hemi-thorax (as it is loculated) without "filling up" the left hemi-thorax.

is often only appreciated on further examination with ultrasound or CT.

Other common causes of benign unilateral, often left-sided, pleural effusions include pancreatitis and post-cardiac bypass surgery. In the latter case they may persist for several weeks postoperatively and it is common to have some residual permanent pleural thickening.

Less common causes include Meigs syndrome (benign ovarian cysts with a left-sided pleural effusion) and yellow nail syndrome.

5.1.2 Bilateral

Benign causes of bilateral pleural effusions are usually associated with particular clinical symptoms and signs that make

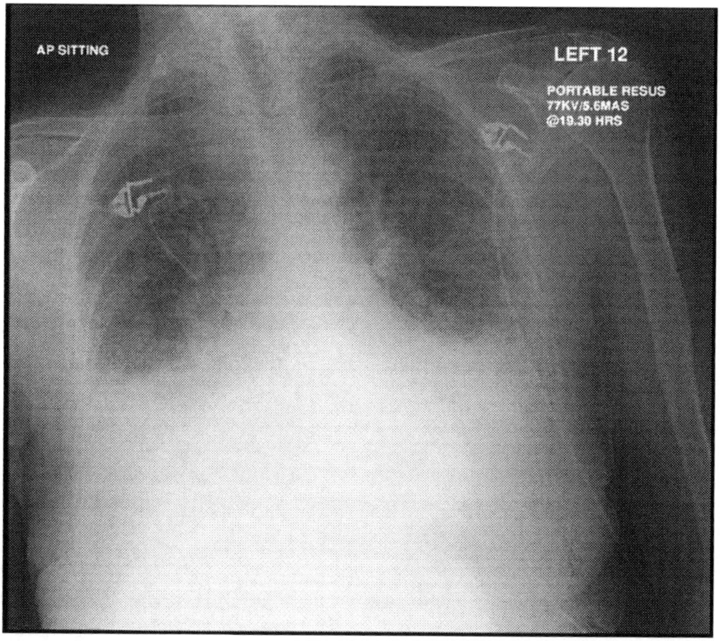

FIGURE 5.5. Left ventricular failure with bilateral pleural effusions.

diagnosis easier, often precluding the need for further specific investigation of the effusion.

Examples include left ventricular failure, chronic renal failure, hypoalbuminemia and ascites.

The associated radiological features of left ventricular failure are cardiac enlargement, perihilar reticulation, and diffuse ground glass opacity as well as the presence of pleural effusions (Fig. 5.5).

5.2 Malignant Pleural Effusions

5.2.1 Unilateral

Unilateral effusions may reflect an underlying malignancy and therefore if there is no obvious evidence of infection or

a

b

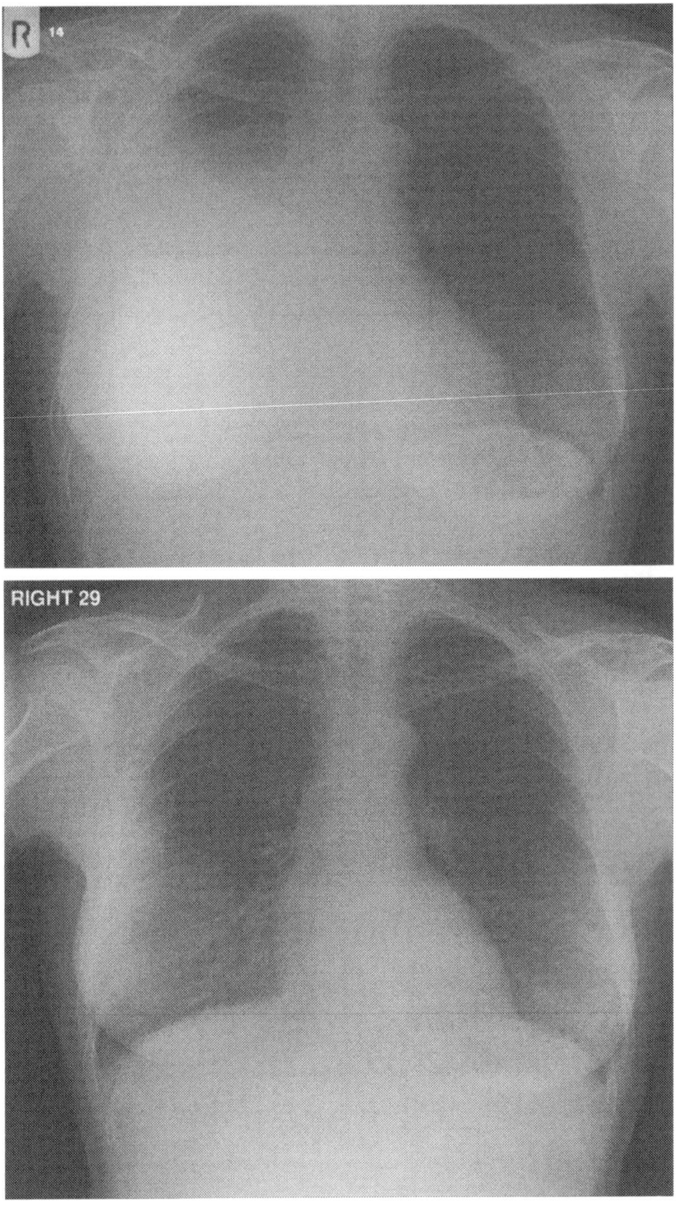

FIGURE 5.6. Right pleural metastatic effusion before (a) and after (b) drainage in a patient with metastatic breast carcinoma. The peripheral pleural metastases are now visible. Note right breast implant.

infarction, they need to be followed up to resolution or investigated further. A large or moderate unilateral effusion will need to be tapped and ideally drained to allow further investigation with either repeat plain film or CT. Drainage allows the underlying lung and pleura, which was initially obscured by the fluid, to be examined (Fig. 5.6a and b).

A malignant effusion may appear benign, but there are some radiological clues that are suggestive of a malignancy.

Volume loss associated with an effusion suggests malignancy until proved otherwise. This is caused by the circumferential contracting nature of pleural malignancy, be it due to pleural metastatic disease or primary disease, such as mesothelioma. Pleural masses or thickening may also suggest malignancy as do the presence of bone or lung metastases.

5.2.2 Bilateral

Malignant effusions are less commonly bilateral, unless there are, for example, multiple pleural metastases. It is very unusual to have bilateral primary pleural malignancy.

5.3 Key Points

1) Unilateral effusions require follow-up and further investigation.
2) Drainage of a unilateral effusion may reveal the underlying pathology.
3) Volume loss associated with an effusion suggests malignancy.

Chapter 5b
Pleural Thickening and Calcification

It can sometimes be difficult to distinguish pleural thickening from an effusion purely on a plain film, particularly when the degree of thickening is small. As mentioned before, comparison with previous imaging or assessment with ultrasound is very useful.

The significance of the thickening may be trivial or serious depending on its cause. Thickening results in opacification that continues up the wall of the hemi-thorax in a way that gravity would not allow an effusion to behave unless loculated. This means that for the degree of pleural opacification, it can track higher than one would expect an effusion to.

In Fig. 5.7 there is pleural thickening tracking toward the midzone. In this case there is also a small amount of volume loss due to scarring and associated contraction. A pleural effusion causing this degree of opacification would remain in the bases (assuming the patient is upright).

Pleural opacification reaching the apex of the thorax in an erect patient is more suggestive of thickening than fluid, although in a supine patient apical fluid can be seen as detailed previously.

The exception to this rule would be a loculated effusion as is sometimes demonstrated in an empyema. However, the degree of density, opacification, and irregularity of a loculated pleural effusion would be greater.

There are both benign and malignant causes for pleural thickening. We will give examples of both separately.

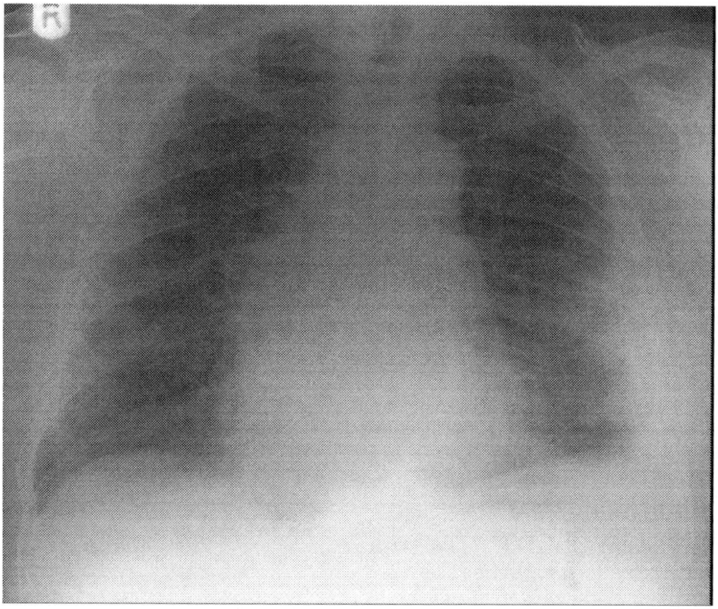

FIGURE 5.7. Benign pleural thickening.

5.4 Benign Pleural Thickening

In general any scarring of the pleura from previous insult may appear in time as thickening. This is commonly due to a previous infection or infarction; other causes include trauma resulting in hemorrhagic effusions or thoracic surgery. A plaque related to asbestos exposure may simply appear as an area of thickening, but calcification is common. Prior radiotherapy can cause pleural thickening localized to the radiation field and there may be accompanying parenchymal changes of fibrosis or atelectasis. In general there is unlikely to be significant volume loss with benign pleural thickening. The exception to this is any condition causing extensive scarring, such as a previous empyema or surgery (Fig. 5.8). The presence of significant volume loss should alert the reader to the possibility of a more sinister cause.

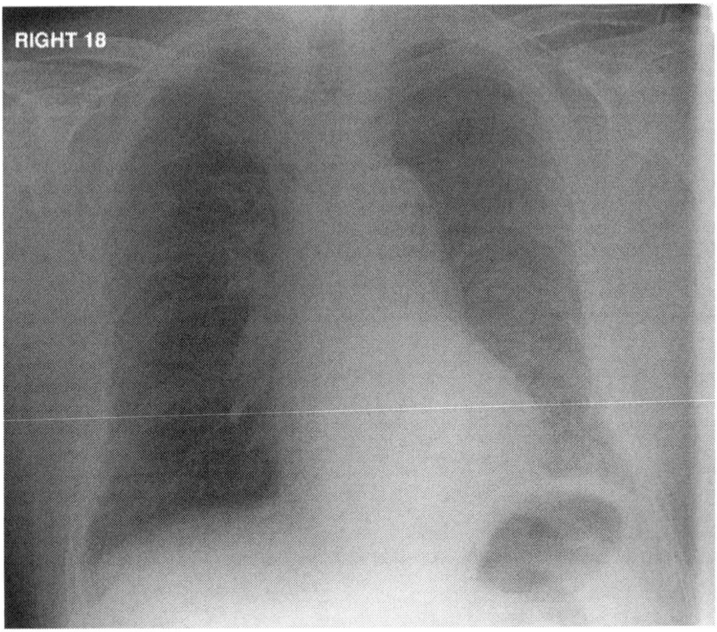

FIGURE 5.8. Pleural thickening post-empyema.

Focal pleural thickening can also be due to a benign pleural fibroma. The appearance of these remains static over multiple films, but the diagnosis is, however, often made upon biopsy.

5.5 Benign Pleural Thickening with Calcification

Calcification is generally a reassuring sign as it suggests a chronic condition. Pleural thickening associated with calcification is seen after infections that involve the pleura, most commonly tuberculosis. There are often other signs such as calcified granulomata, a previous surgical thoracoplasty, or lobectomy and sometimes pneumonectomy (Fig. 5.9). Again the appearances are often stable in comparison with previous films. Pleural calcification typically produces sheets or

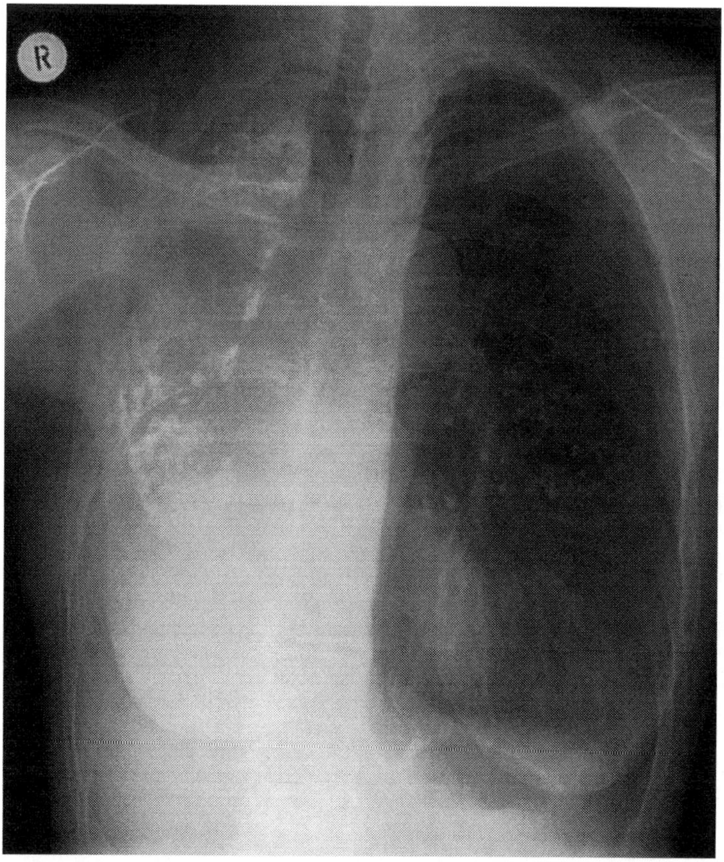

FIGURE 5.9. Pneumonectomy and pleural calcification (old TB). There is a "sheet" of pleural calcification and mediastinal shift to the right filling the "space" created by the pneumonectomy. On the left there are multiple parenchymal calcified granulomata.

"flat areas" that do not conform to the normal outlines of parenchymal structures.

Asbestos exposure can result in pleural plaques which often affect the hemi-diaphragms. They can, however, be found anywhere along the pleural surface. Around 50% of these will calcify. When seen "enface" they may have a typical "holly leaf" appearance (Fig. 5.10).

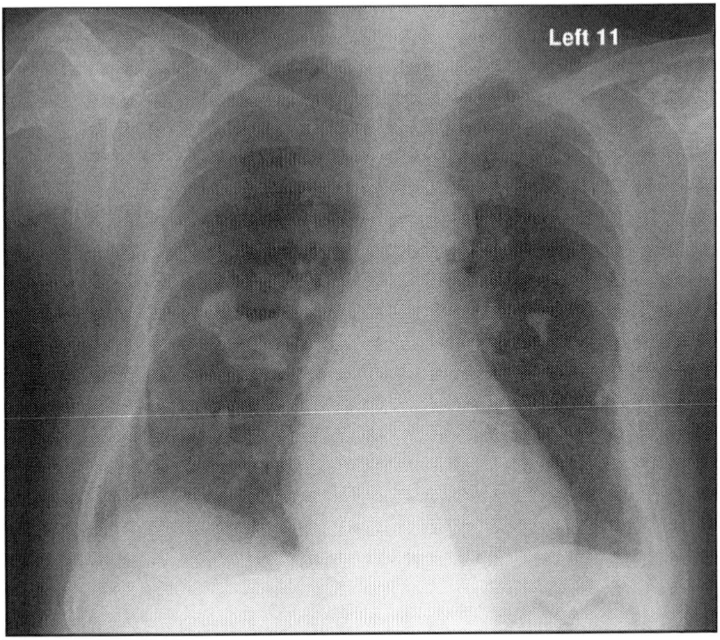

FIGURE 5.10. Holly leaf calcification following asbestos exposure.

5.6 Malignant Pleural Thickening

The two main pathologies to consider are mesothelioma and pleural metastases.

The clues to malignancy are in general progressive disease, volume loss, and involvement of the mediastinal pleura. If extensive disease is present, there may be a rind of pleural thickening encircling the lungs causing constriction and therefore volume loss (Fig. 5.11). This sign is particularly well seen on CT, but may be present on the chest X-ray, particularly if looked for. There may be associated pleural effusions.

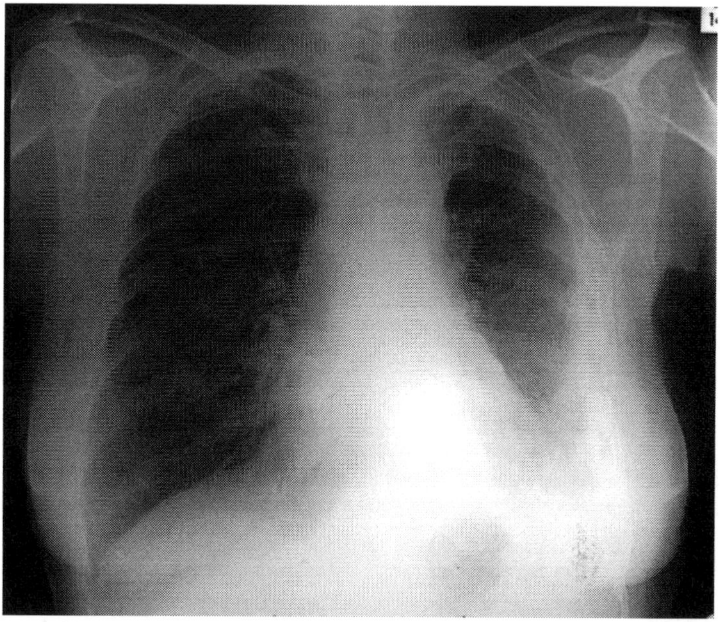

FIGURE 5.11. Mesothelioma.

Pleural metastases are most commonly from a lung or breast primary. In this example there is a left hilar bronchogenic carcinoma and multiple pleural metastases (Fig. 5.12).

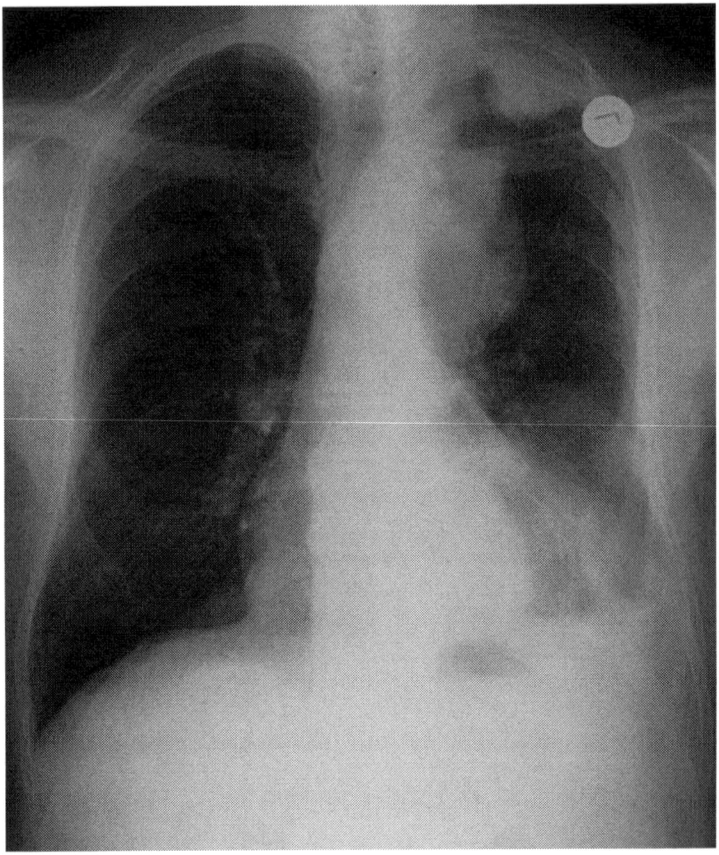

FIGURE 5.12. Pleural metastases from a left hilar bronchogenic carcinoma.

5.7 Key Points

1) Benign pleural thickening remains unchanged on comparison with previous films.
2) Calcification within areas of thickening usually suggests a benign cause.
3) Malignant pleural thickening is commonly associated with volume loss.
4) Ultrasound is useful to differentiate between pleural thickening and an effusion.

Chapter 5c
Pneumothorax

The confident diagnosis of a pneumothorax is a good example of an abnormality that may cause a diagnostic challenge to a junior doctor. There is clearly significance to the diagnosis as intervention in the form of a chest drain may be required.

The diagnosis may be very easy in the context of significant trauma with appropriate symptoms and the presence of a large pneumothorax on a chest X-ray. More commonly, however, the presenting symptom may simply be shortness of breath, for which there are clearly many causes and the appearances on the chest X-ray may be very subtle. We will give in this section an approach to interpretation that should make confident diagnosis much easier.

The key sign is asymmetrical loss of lung markings accompanied by a visible margin. This new margin representing the edge of the lung is seen as the pneumothorax results in a new soft tissue/air interface (Fig. 5.13).

There are other causes of asymmetrical loss of lung marking such as emphysema and the normal ageing process of the lungs. It is very important therefore to identify the new margin created by the lung edge. Attributing loss of lung markings alone to a pneumothorax will result in overdiagnosis. The presence of bullae can result in misinterpretation, with the inner aspect of a bulla being incorrectly identified as the lung edge. In these cases, however, the "line" seen would be focal rather than extending over a reasonable length of the hemithorax (Fig. 5.14). Comparison with old films can in this circumstance be very helpful.

If there is strong clinical suspicion of a pneumothorax that does not appear to be demonstrated, the conspicuity can be

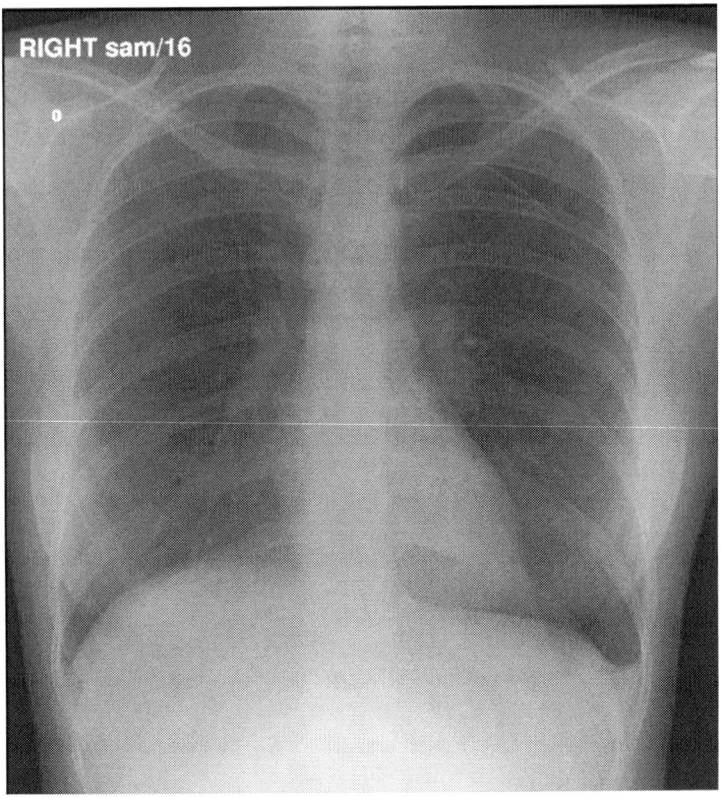

FIGURE 5.13. Left pneumothorax.

increased by performing an expiratory film. A pneumothorax will be larger on an expiratory film, due to the relative decrease in the lung volume compared to an inspiratory film.

Overlying soft tissue folds may also be misinterpreted as a lung edge. This mistake can be avoided by noting that the "line" continues outside the hemi-thorax and therefore cannot be a representation of the lung margin.

Large pneumothoraces can result in significantly increased perfusion of the normal lung as most of the blood is redirected to the "good" side. This lung therefore appears relatively opaque and can be confused with consolidation (Fig. 5.15).

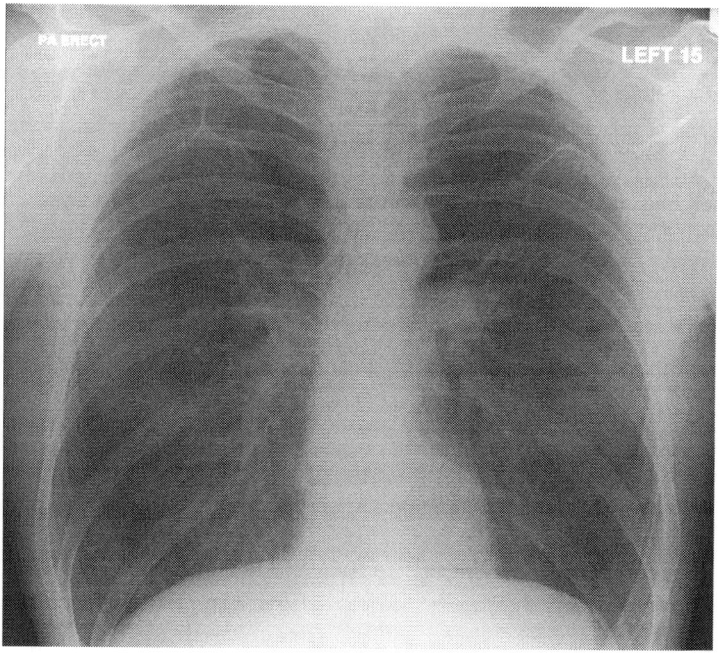

FIGURE 5.14. Apical focal bullae.

Pneumothoraces are traditionally divided into spontaneous and traumatic with a sub-division into primary and secondary. While the full list of causes of pneumothoraces is beyond the scope of this book, the more common will be discussed.

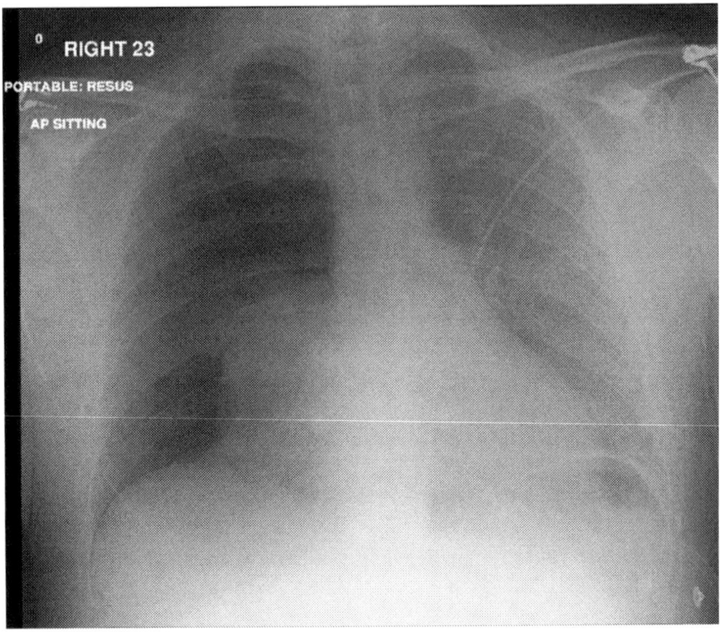

FIGURE 5.15. Large right pneumothorax with increased perfusion left lung.

5.8 Spontaneous

Primary spontaneous pneumothoraces typically occur in tall, thin males.

Secondary causes may be related to underlying chronic lung conditions, such as COPD, asthma, and cystic fibrosis.

5.9 Traumatic

This can be sub-divided into iatrogenic and penetrating. Iatrogenic causes are many, but are particularly common after intervention, such as aspiration of pleural fluid, post-lung biopsy, and pacemaker insertions. In Fig. 5.16 there is in fact a hydropneumothorax due to a small residual effusion

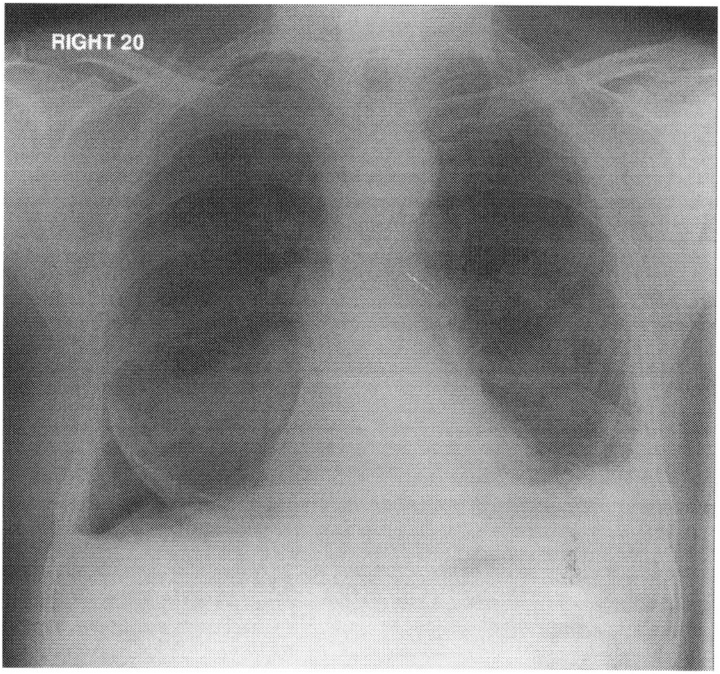

FIGURE 5.16. Right hydropneumothorax following aspiration of pleural effusion.

post-aspiration. Note the air fluid level present. Pneumothorax is a common complication of mechanical ventilation.

Penetrating causes include direct trauma, such as stab wounds, and secondary puncture from fractures of the thoracic cage (Fig. 5.17).

Once a pneumothorax has been identified, it is important to determine whether there is any element of "tension." A tension pneumothorax is a medical emergency. This condition is generally diagnosed clinically and treated promptly, but it is very important to recognize an unsuspected tension pneumothorax that is demonstrated radiographically (Figs. 5.18 and 5.19).

As with all things, pneumothoraces become easier to see with practice and experience. If you consider the possibility of

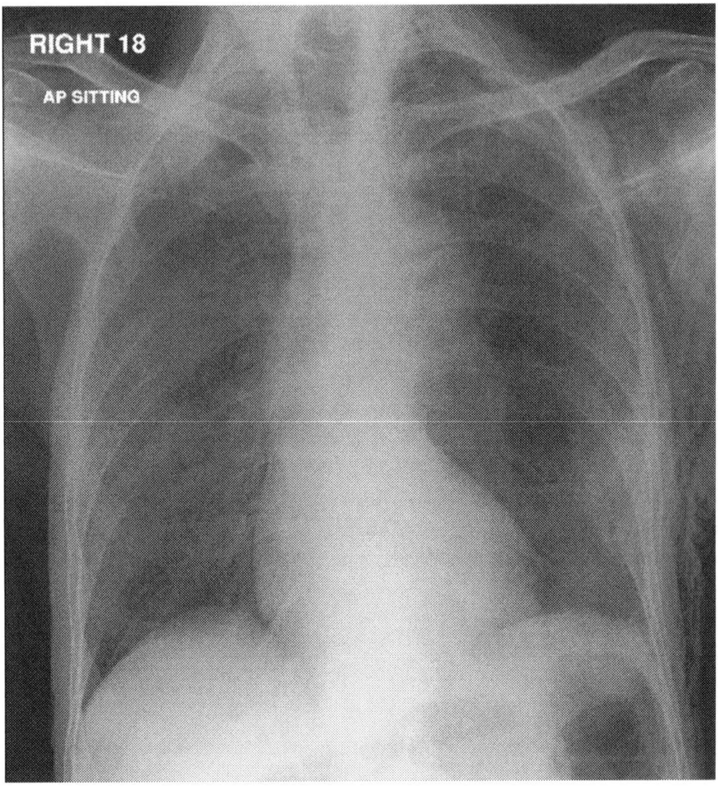

FIGURE 5.17. Fracture of the left posterior seventh and eighth ribs, surgical emphysema, and small left apical pneumothorax.

a pneumothorax whenever you review a chest X-ray, particularly in the appropriate clinical context, you will be unlikely to miss one. The value of comparison with old films should not be underestimated and it will also help avoid pitfalls, such as soft tissue folds and bullae that result in overdiagnosis. Once a pneumothorax has been diagnosed, it is essential to exclude the presence of tension.

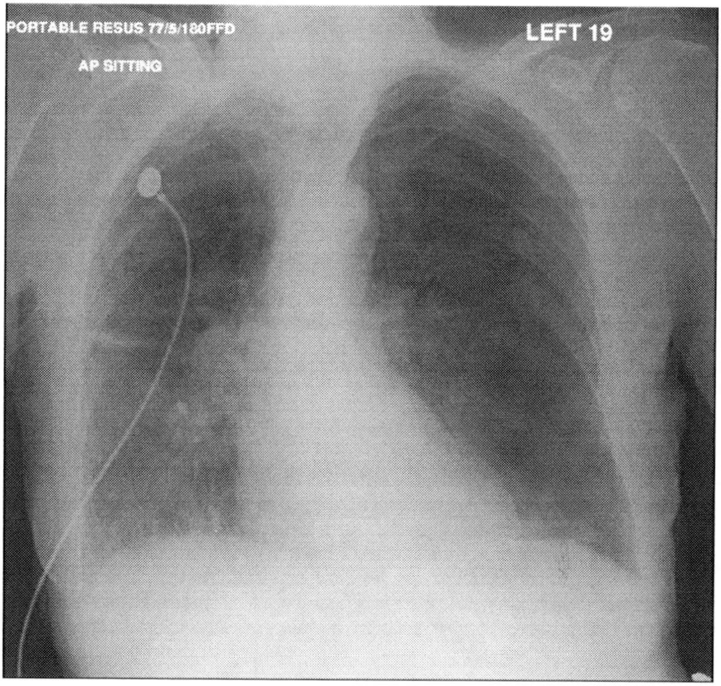

FIGURE 5.18. Left tension pneumothorax with mediastinal shift to the right.

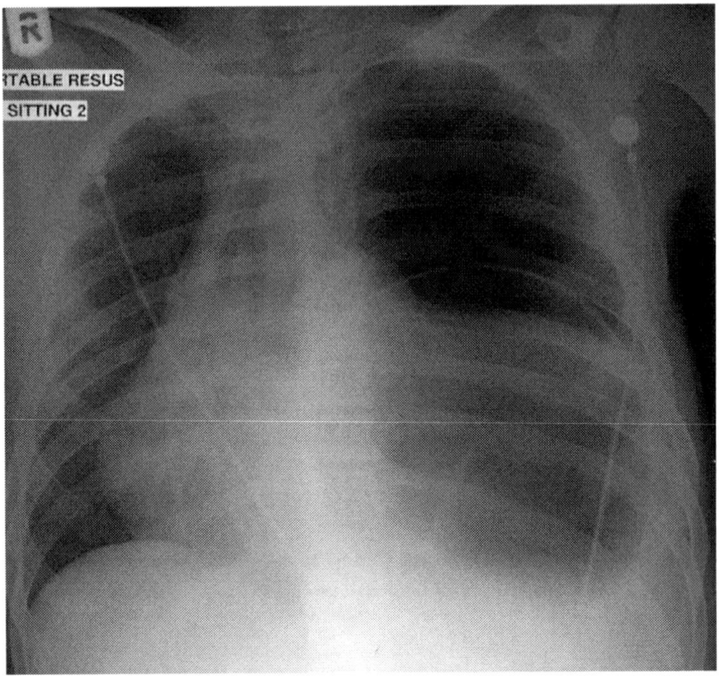

FIGURE 5.19. Left tension pneumothorax with rupture of left hemi-diaphragm and herniation of stomach into left hemi-thorax.

5.10 Key Points

1) Look for loss of lung markings and then for the lung edge.
2) Look for evidence of tension.
3) Expiratory films can make a small pneumothorax easier to identify.
4) Do not confuse skin folds or bullae with pneumothoraces.
5) In the presence of fractured ribs look for a pneumothorax.
6) Large pneumothoraces can result in increased perfusion of other lung.

Chapter 6
Soft Tissues and Bony Structures

When examining a chest X-ray it is very important to consider the peripheral structures. Details of a review of areas have been given in Chapter 2 and we will now return to these as they apply to soft tissue structures and bones.

Making a conscious effort to look at all the specific regions will prevent you from missing an important abnormality or a clue as to the underlying pathology. The important review area in terms of soft tissue include below the diaphragms, the periphery of the chest wall, the supraclavicular region, and neck as far as included on the film (Figs. 6.1, 6.2, and 6.3).

Free air beneath the diaphragm may be the only clue of a silent perforation of an intra-abdominal viscus, for example, in a patient on steroids (Fig. 6.4).

A nodal mass within the neck may not have been felt on clinical examination, but may be visible on the chest X-ray. Further review areas should include the breast shadows, the shoulders, and the bony structures of the thoracic cage, such as the ribs and thoracic spine (Figs. 6.5, 6.6, and 6.7).

Many soft tissues and bony abnormalities that appear on the chest X-ray are likely to be quickly apparent to an examining clinician, but these areas may not have been examined before the review of the chest X-ray. The presence, for example, of a mastectomy should alert you to other possibilities such as a metastases or a recurrence of previous carcinomas.

R. Joarder, N. Crundwell (eds.), *Chest X-Ray in Clinical Practice*,
DOI 10.1007/978-1-84882-099-9_6,

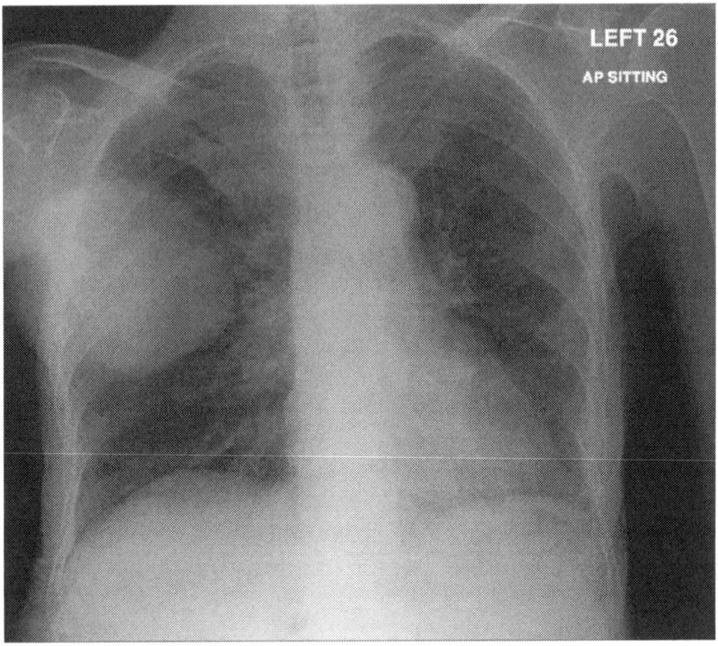

FIGURE 6.1. Right chest wall sarcoma.

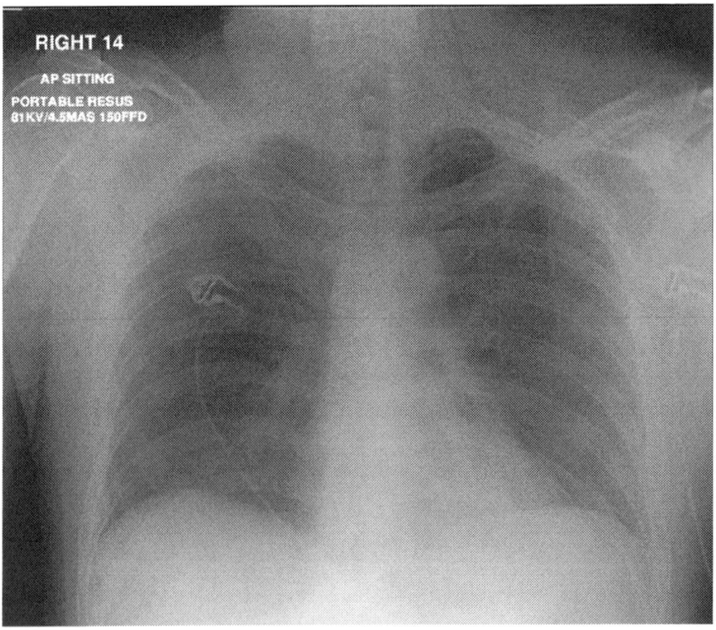

FIGURE 6.2. Left supraclavicular surgical emphysema.

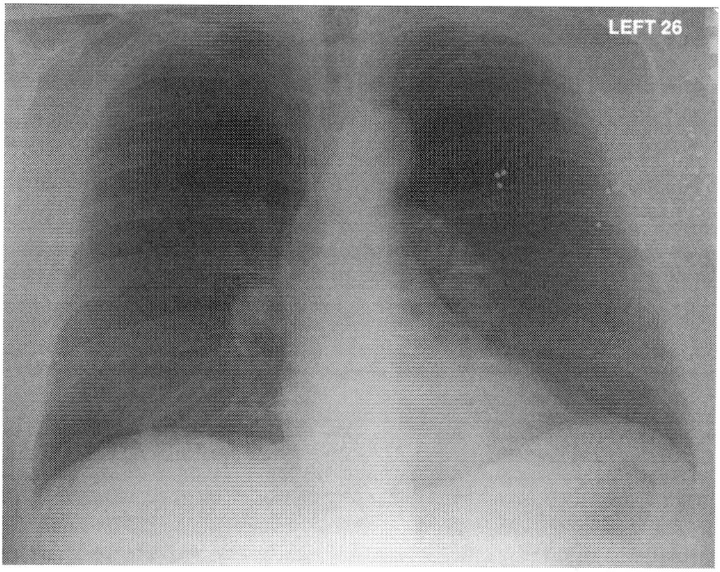

FIGURE 6.3. Old gunshot wound.

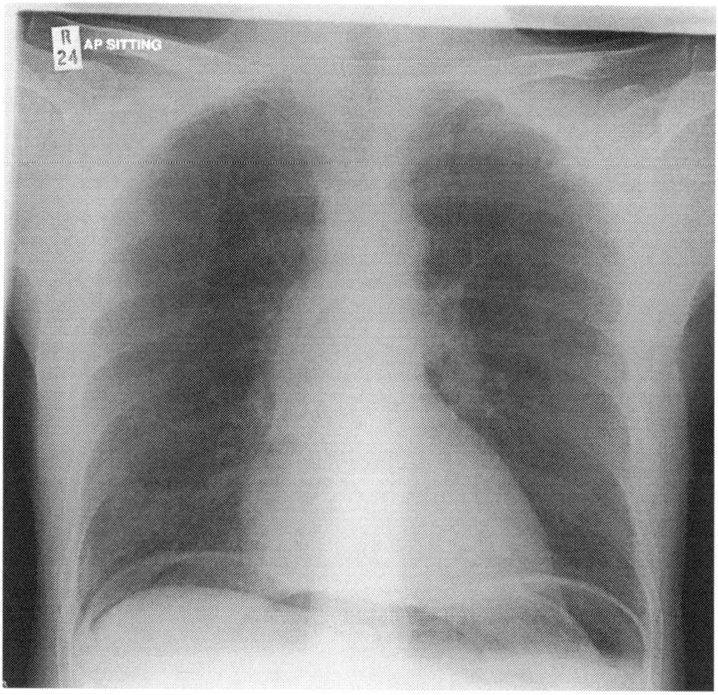

FIGURE 6.4. Free air beneath both hemi-diaphragms. Note the continuous diaphragm crossing midline.

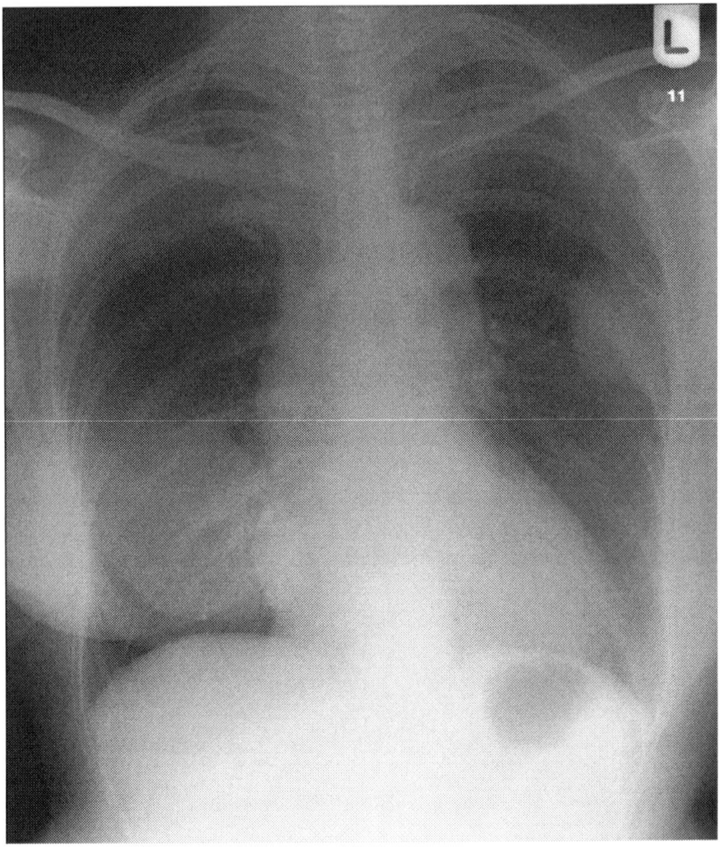

FIGURE 6.5. Left sixth rib neurofibroma, note the rib notching.

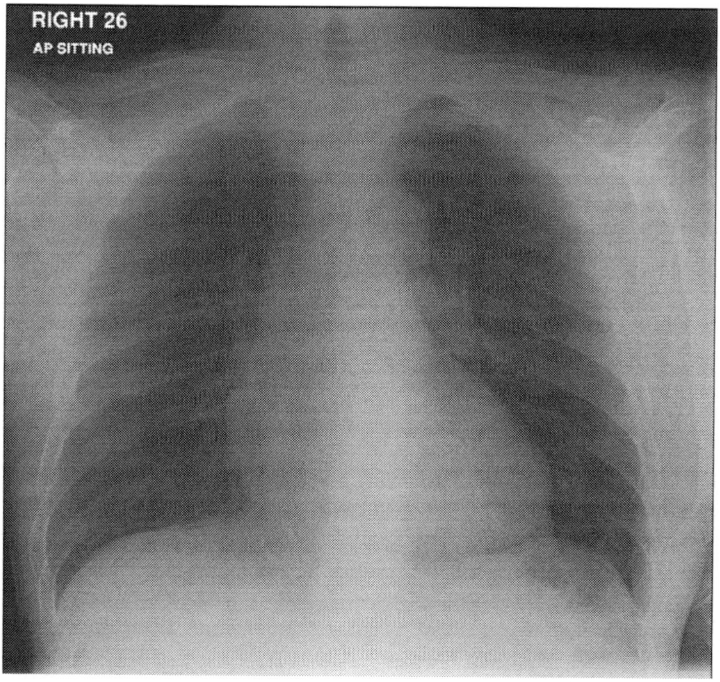

FIGURE 6.6. Fracture of the distal left clavicle.

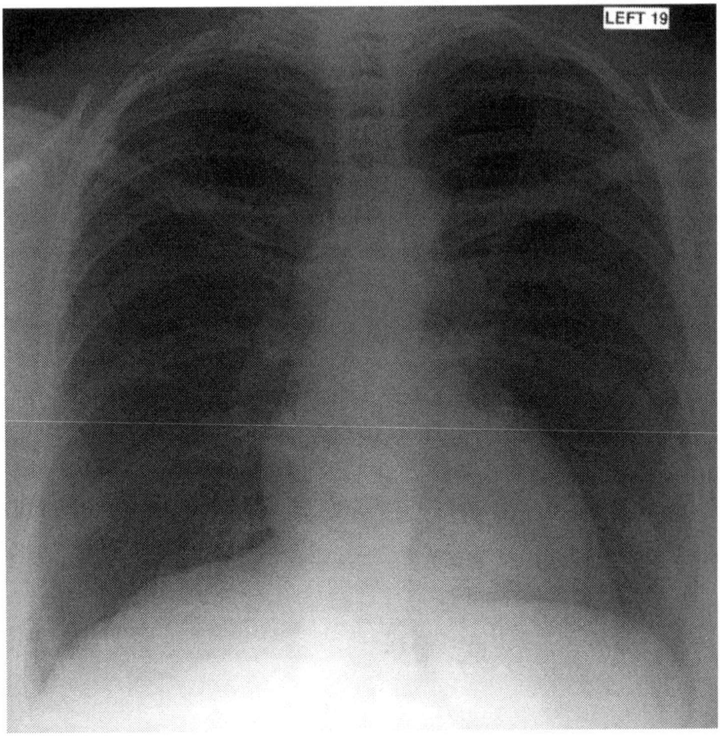

FIGURE 6.7. Right cervical rib.

A swallowed or ingested foreign body may not always be volunteered by the patient, for example, psychiatric patients or young children (Fig. 6.8). Other more exotic swallowed substances include drug-filled packages.

There can be particular associations with bony abnormalities. Generally sclerotic bones may be an indication of a metastatic prostate cancer (Fig. 6.9) and generally lucent bones may relate to myeloma. Erosion of the medial aspects of the clavicles occurs in rheumatoid arthritis. This can be associated with benign lung nodules. The bones may appear coarse and expanded in Paget's disease (Fig. 6.10). Ankylosing spondylitis will result in a bamboo spine as well as apical fibrosis.

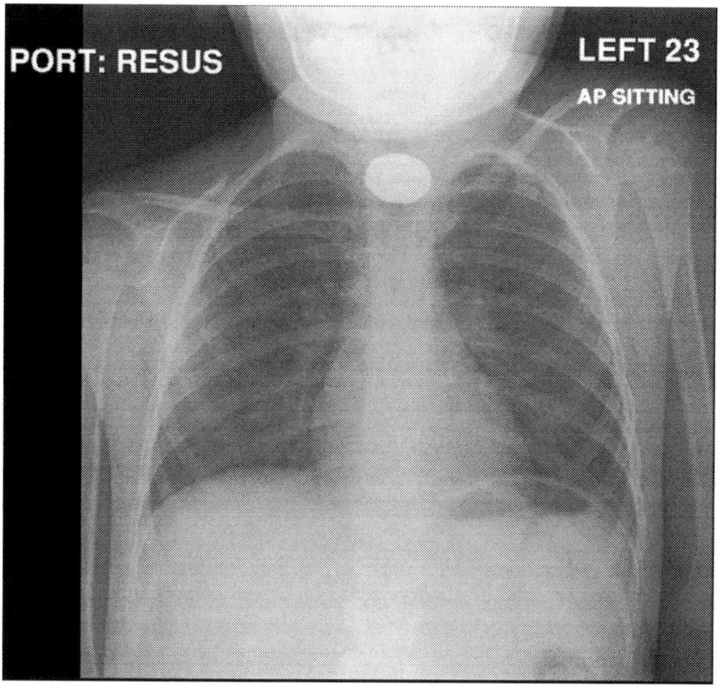

FIGURE 6.8. Swallowed 20 pence piece.

It is in general harder to spot an abnormality that is the result of an absence of a structure than the presence. This is particularly true of soft tissues or bony structures. It is, however, extremely important to identify missing ribs as these may be the only indication of an adjacent neoplastic lesion, which may be primary or the result of a metastatic disease (Figs. 6.11, 6.12, and 6.13).

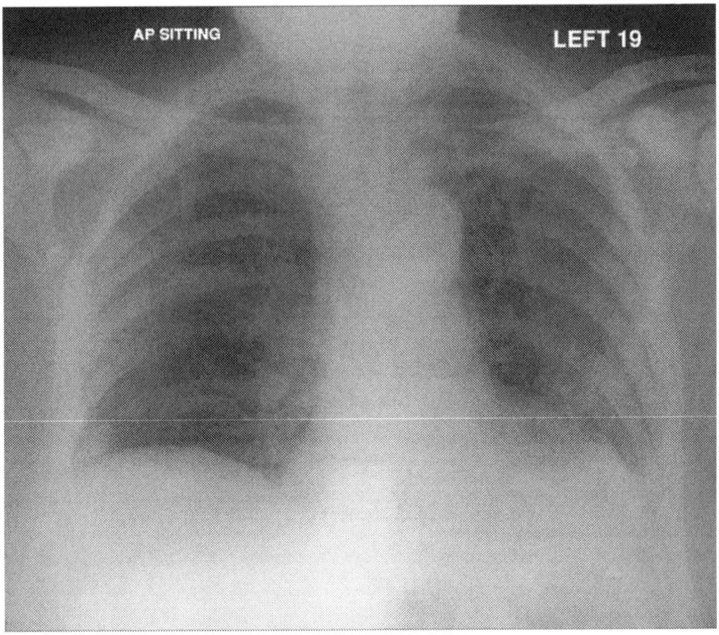

FIGURE 6.9. Sclerotic bony metastases from prostate cancer.

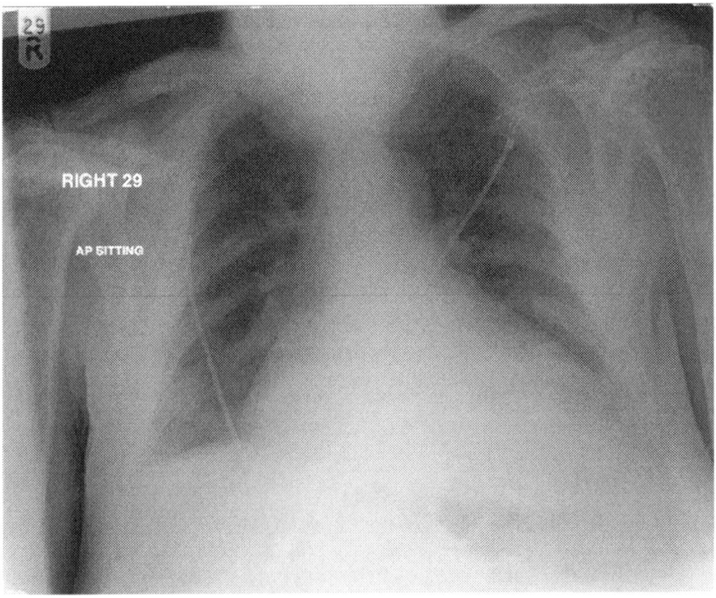

FIGURE 6.10. Paget's left humerus, clavicle, and scapula.

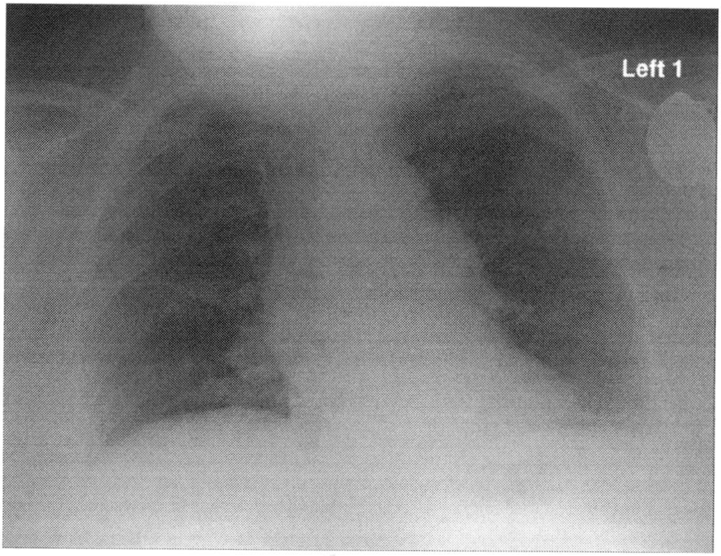

FIGURE 6.11. Missing left posterior fifth rib.

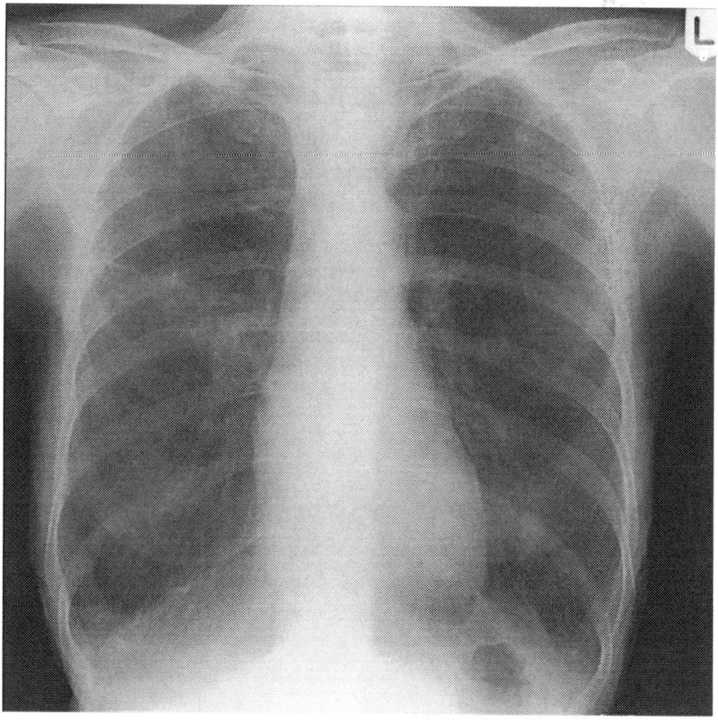

FIGURE 6.12. Missing right posterior fifth rib with bulky right hilum.

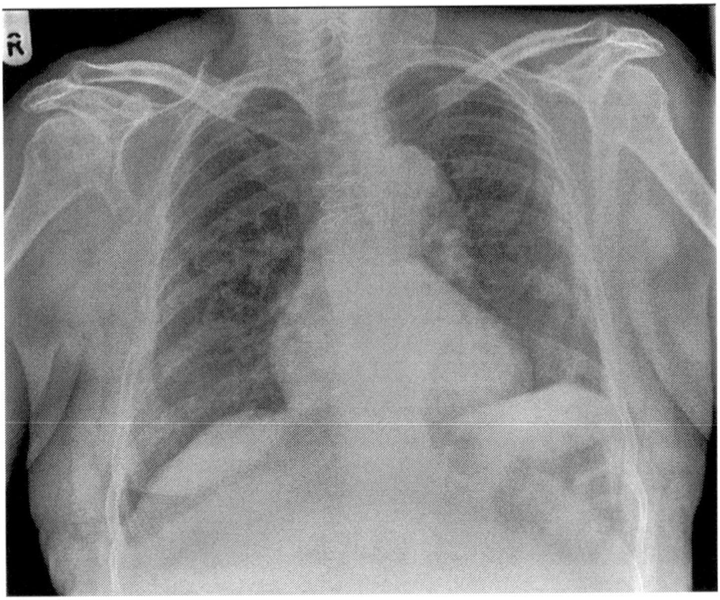

FIGURE 6.13. Missing inferior half right scapula from a sarcoma.

6.1 Key Points

1) Always check your review areas.
2) Missing structures are easy to overlook but have a high significance.

Chapter 7
Foreign Structures and Other Devices on Chest X-rays

There are a variety of other findings on chest X-rays that relate to either previous surgical procedures or line/tube placement. This chapter gives a range of examples that may be useful.

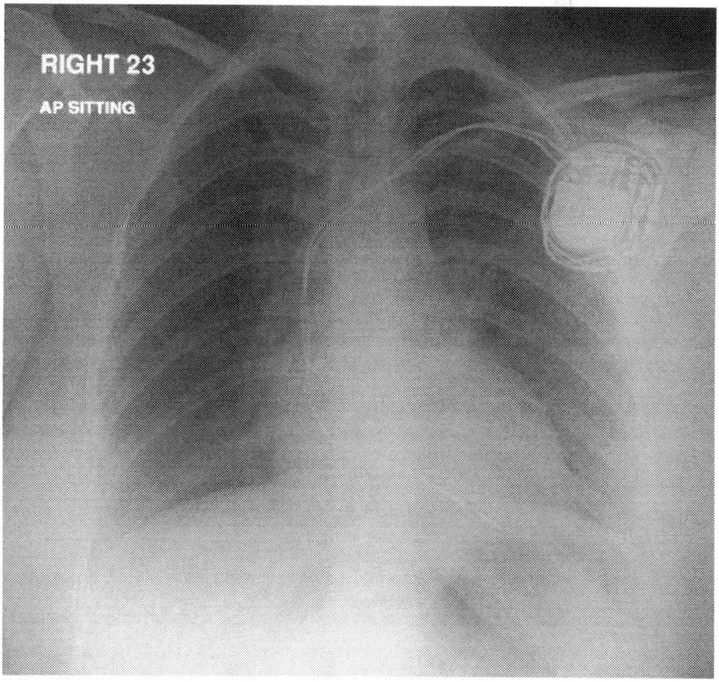

FIGURE 7.1. Dual chamber permanent pacemaker.

R. Joarder, N. Crundwell (eds.), *Chest X-Ray in Clinical Practice*,
DOI 10.1007/978-1-84882-099-9_7,

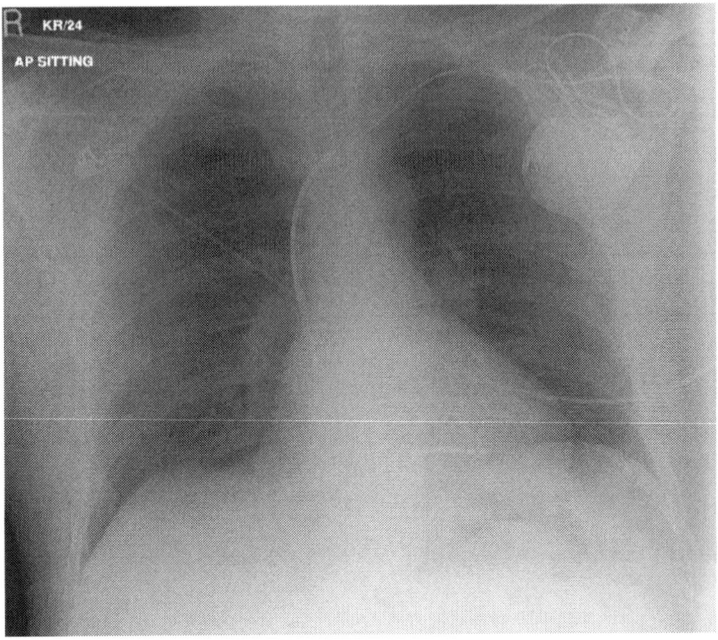

FIGURE 7.2. Internal defibrillator device, note thicker wires than the pacemaker.

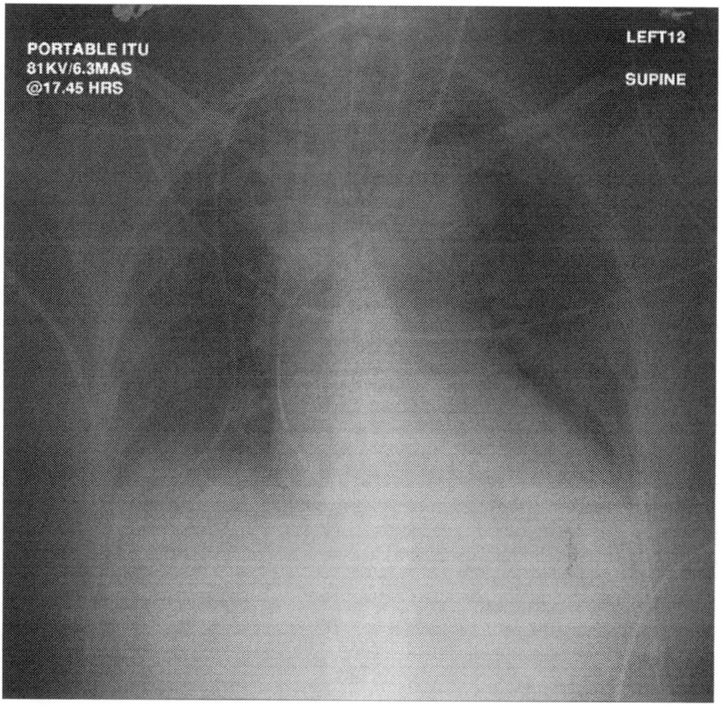

FIGURE 7.3. Temporary external pacemaker within the left internal jugular vein.

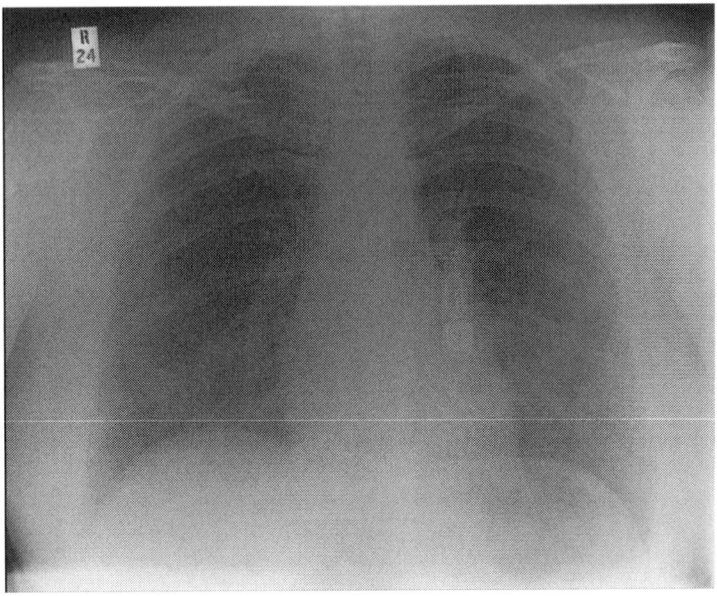

FIGURE 7.4. Reveal device.

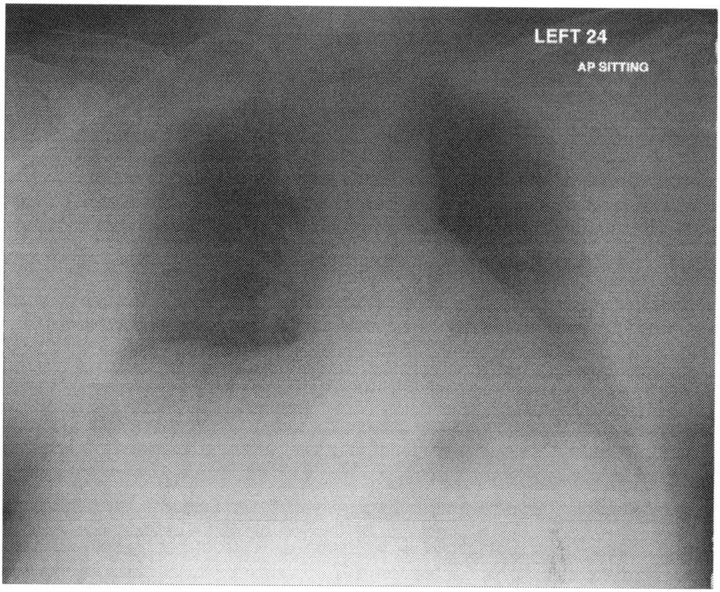

FIGURE 7.5. Vascath.

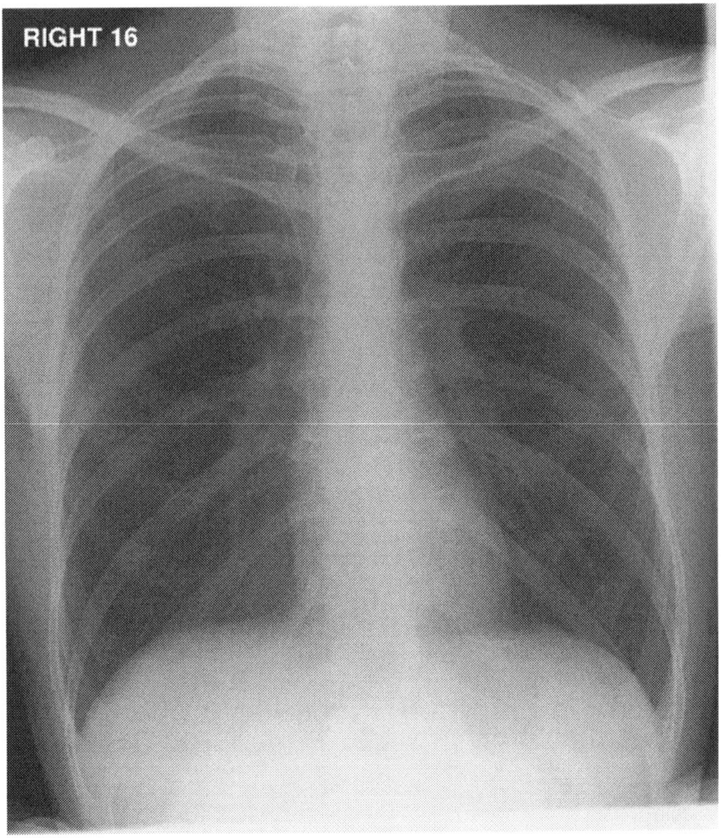

FIGURE 7.6. Peripherally inserted central catheter, the tip is within the right atrium.

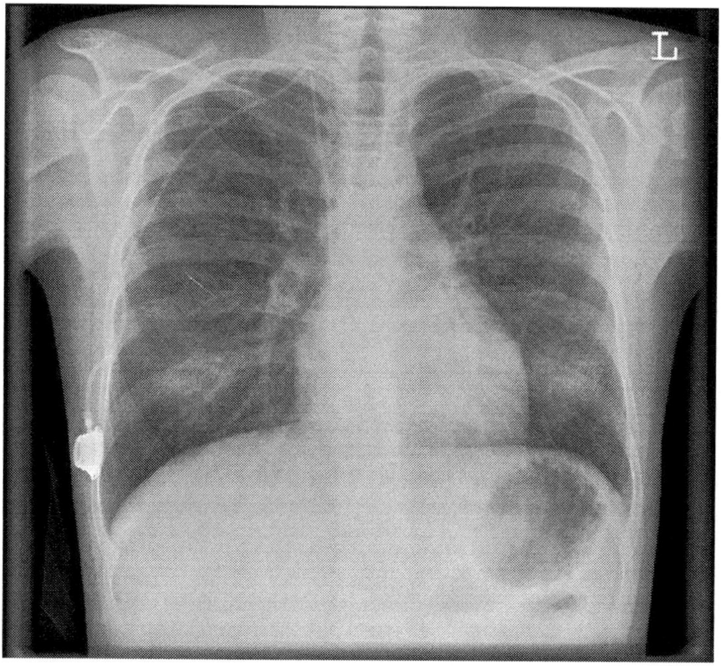

FIGURE 7.7. Portacath in a patient with cystic fibrosis.

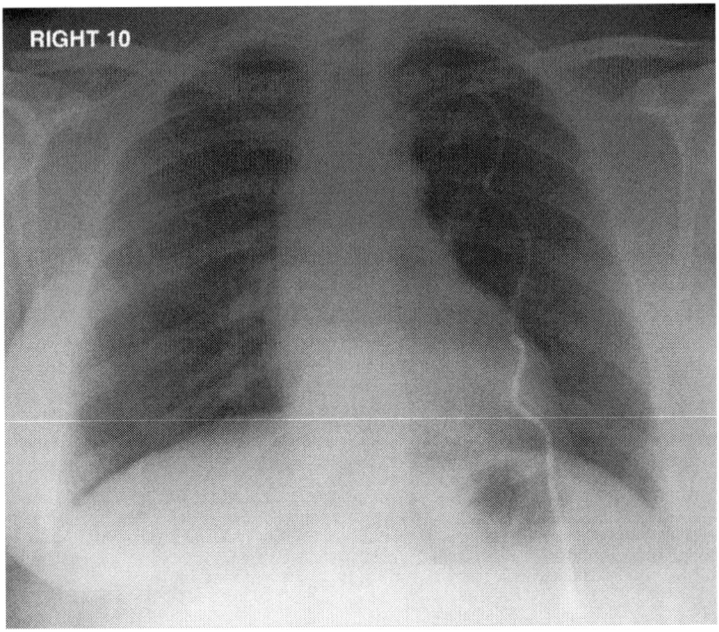

FIGURE 7.8. Hickman line.

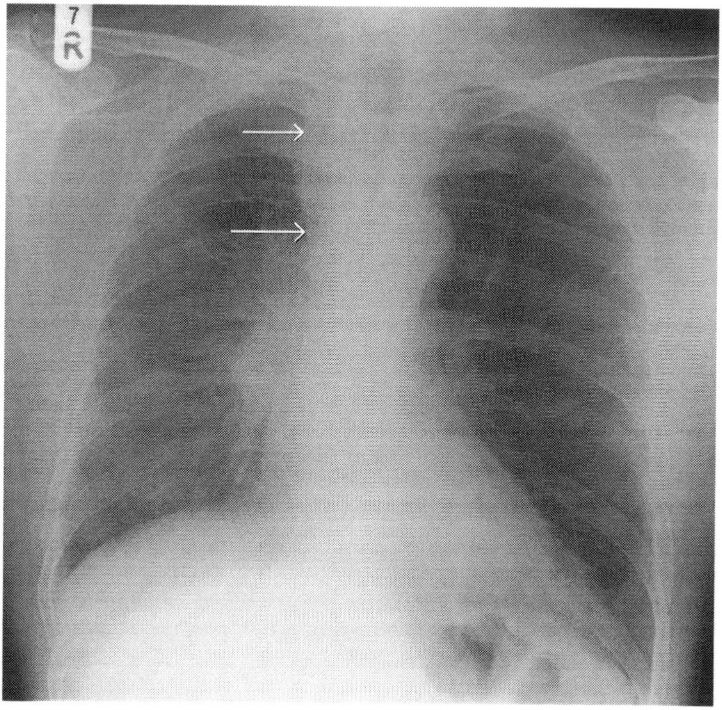

FIGURE 7.9. Superior vena cava stent (*arrows*) in a patient with small cell lung cancer.

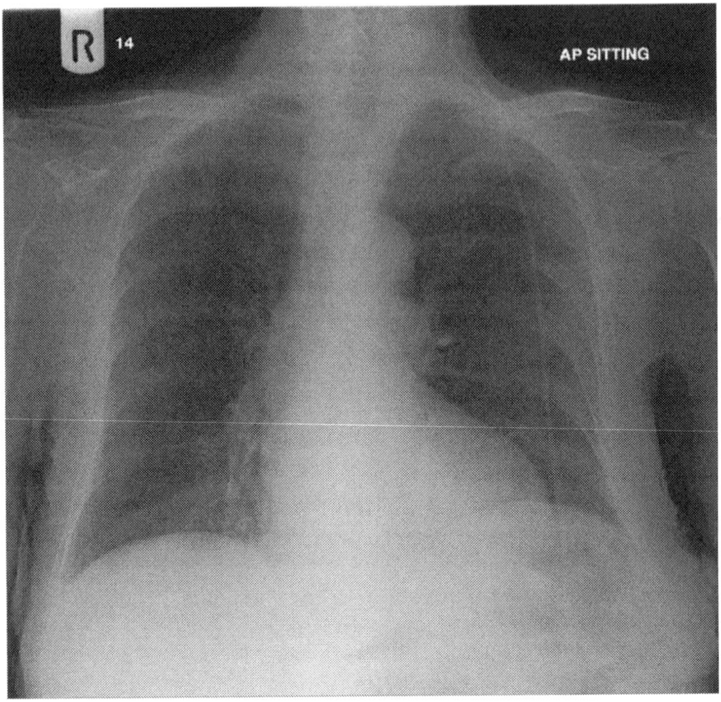

FIGURE 7.10. Ventriculoperitoneal shunt; note this extends from the region of the neck to below the diaphragm.

a

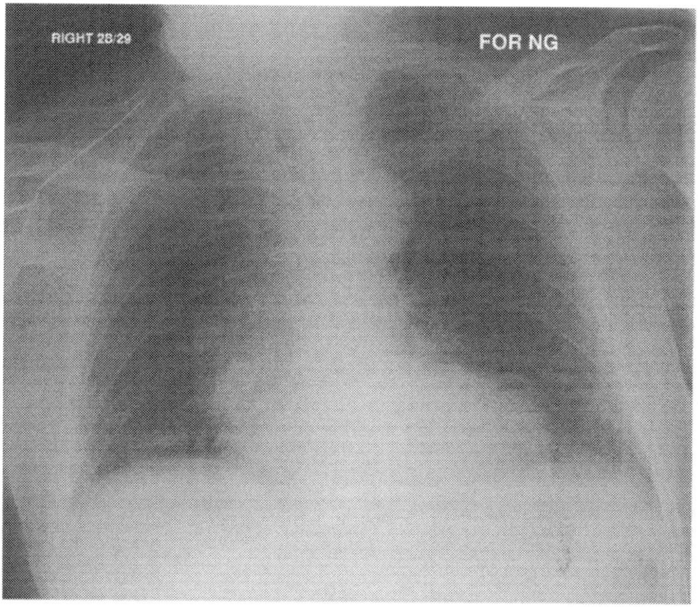

FIGURE 7.11a. Nasogastric tube coiled within the oesophagus.

b

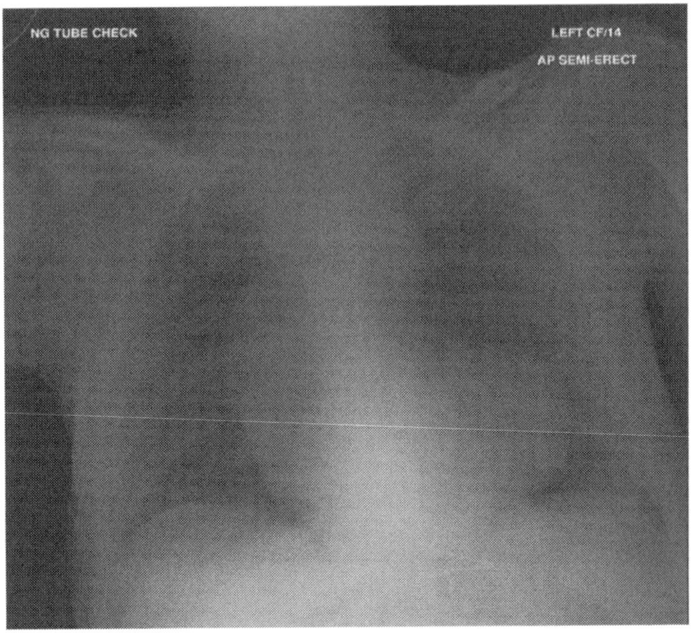

FIGURE 7.11b. Nasogastric tube with tip in the stomach.

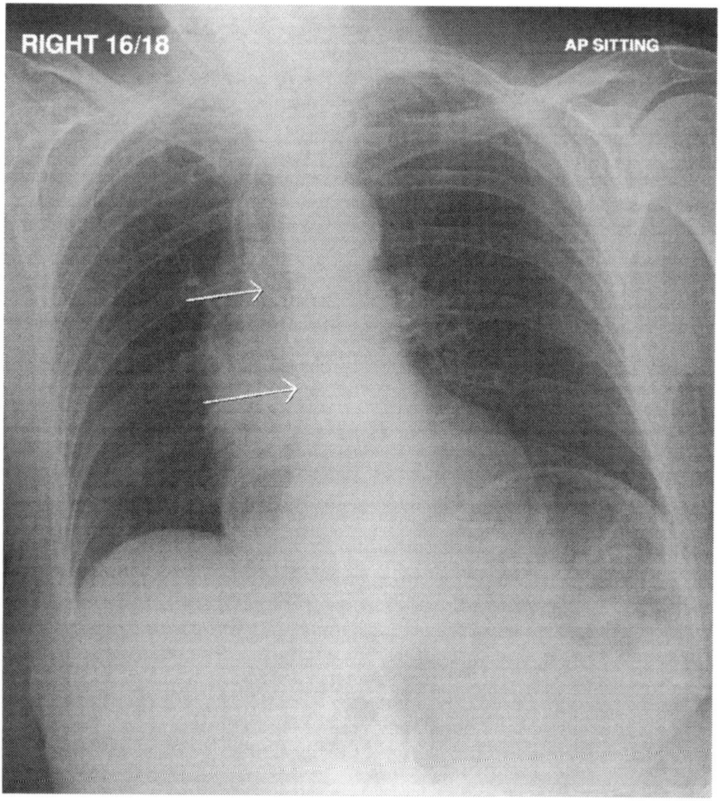

FIGURE 7.12. Oesophageal stent (*arrows*) in a patient with oesophageal carcinoma.

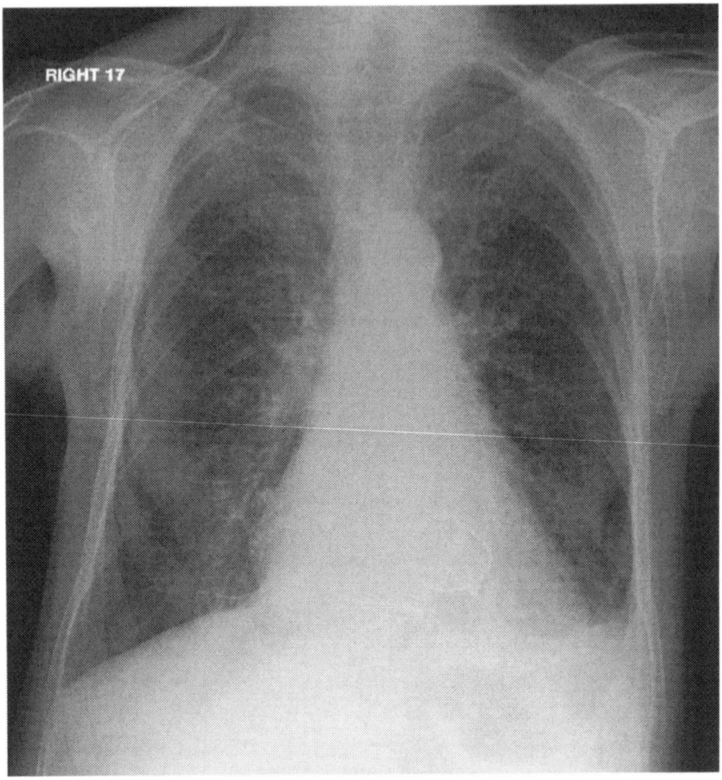

FIGURE 7.13. Mitral valve replacement (metal).

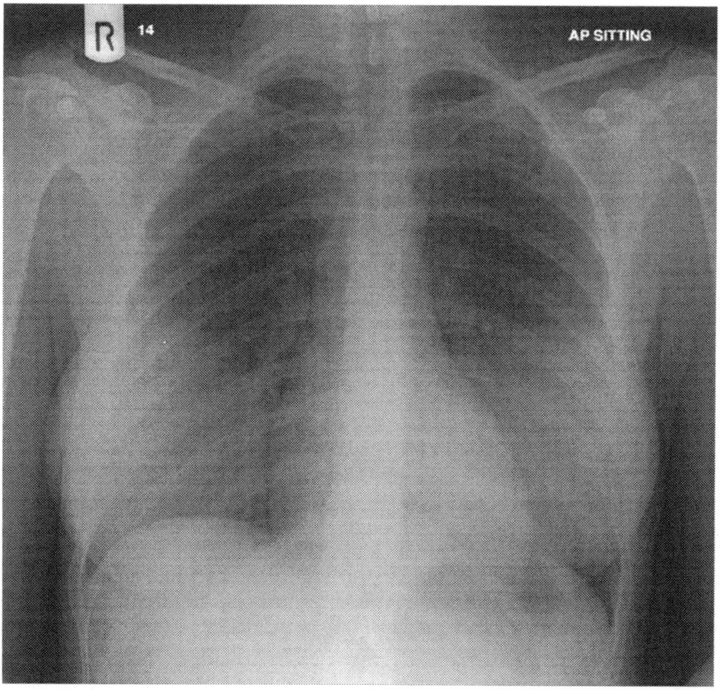

FIGURE 7.14. Bilateral breast implants.

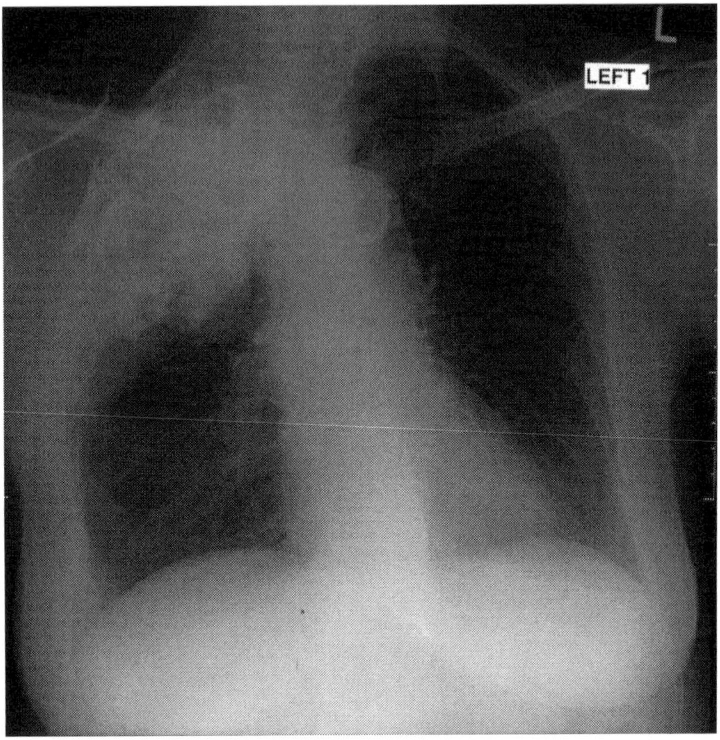

FIGURE 7.15. Right apical plombage (old treatment for TB).

Part III

Chapter 8
Computed Tomography: Technical Information

Computerized tomography (CT) is the name given to an imaging technique in which an X-ray tube and a series of X-ray detectors lie opposite one another in a fixed geometry. The whole mechanism (Fig. 8.1)rotates around the patient, often at very high velocity, while an X-ray exposure is made (the word tomography derives from the Greek *tomos* which means slice or layer and *graphy* which means a representation of a specified object).

By mathematically interpreting the data acquired, the density of each voxel (volume element) of the patient within the scanned area is calculated and assigned a number – the Hounsfield unit (HU) which is also known as the CT number. This value should be directly proportional to the actual voxel density and should also be a constant, i.e., if the same piece of tissue was scanned in another CT scanner, the Hounsfield value should be identical, all other things being equal. This CT value is then assigned to the corresponding pixel (picture element) within the displayed image and a gray scale applied to give a representative display of the densities within the tissue scanned.

The Hounsfield scale is based around a set value of zero for water with tissues of increasing density being allocated higher numbers and those with lower densities being given lower or negative values. Hence, the soft tissues of the liver are around 30–50 HU, blood around 80 HU, and dense compact bone ranging from 1500 to 4000 HU plus. Fat is approximately −90 HU and air is around −1000 depending

R. Joarder, N. Crundwell (eds.), *Chest X-Ray in Clinical Practice*,
DOI 10.1007/978-1-84882-099-9_8,

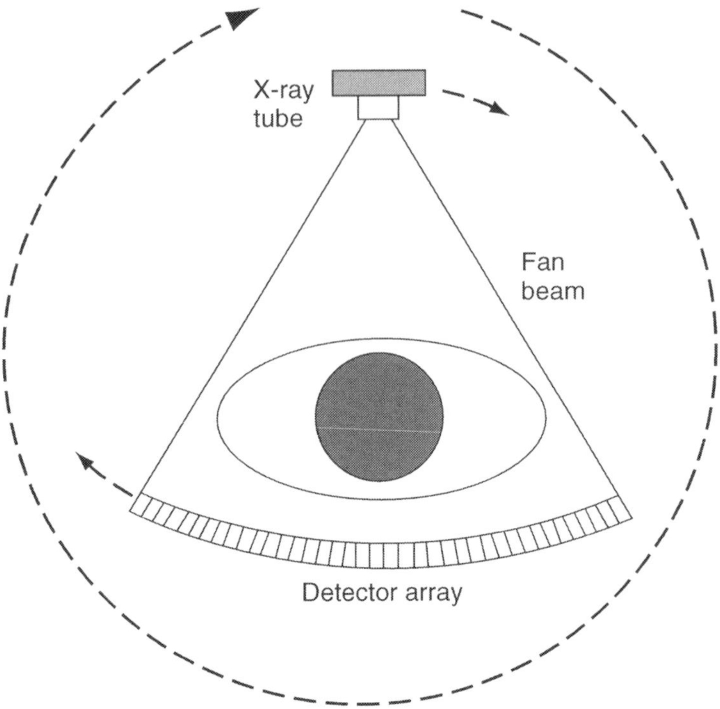

Figure 8.1. Diagram of the geometry of a CT tube and detector array.

upon the barometric pressure at the time of scanning. By using the HU value of tissues within the image, it is possible to help differentiate differing tissues and/or pathologies. There is, however, quite a lot of overlap in HU values between differing soft tissues and so use of these values can only be used as an aid to diagnosis and not a definitive tool.

Early CT scanners acquired a single "slice" of data before moving the patient couch a certain distance and acquiring another slice. Through advances in technology it then became possible for CT scanners to acquire a spiral of data by moving the patient slowly through the scanner while continuously exposing them to X-rays. The latest scanners now use separate rows of detectors to acquire multiple simultaneous spirals of data, i.e., multislice CT (MSCT). This has made the machines much faster with whole chest, abdomen, and pelvis scans being achievable in just a few seconds (Fig. 8.2).

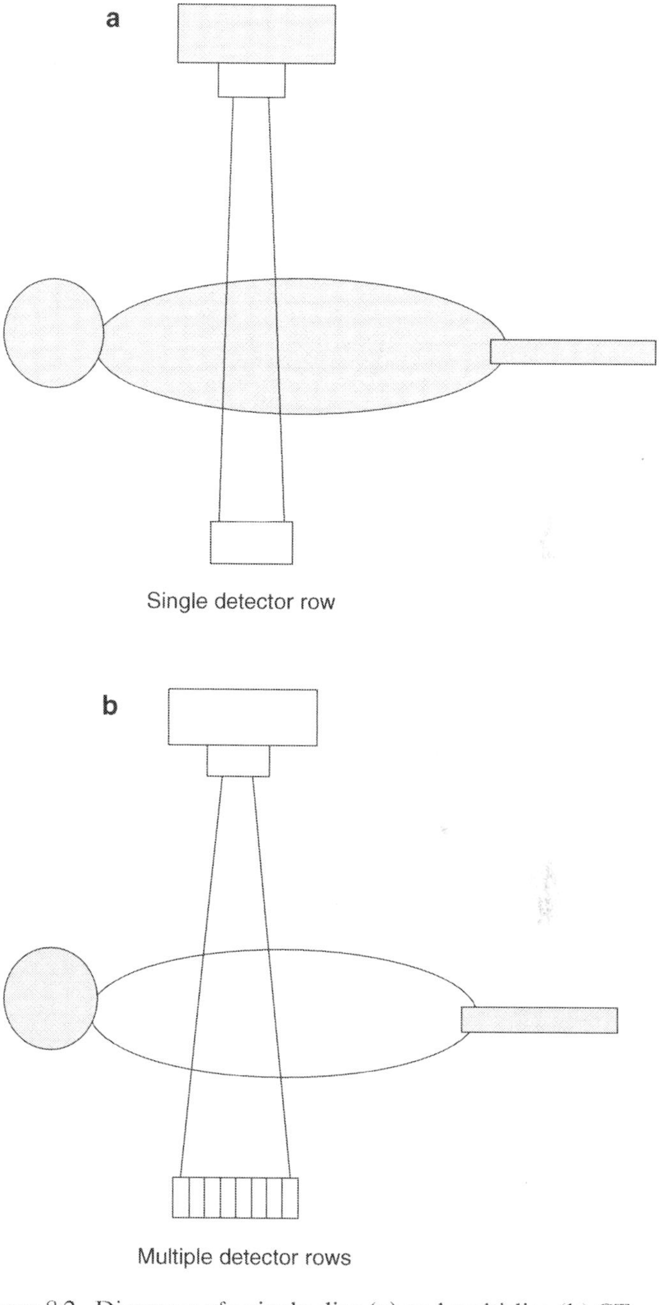

FIGURE 8.2. Diagrams of a single slice (a) and multislice (b) CT scanners in cross section.

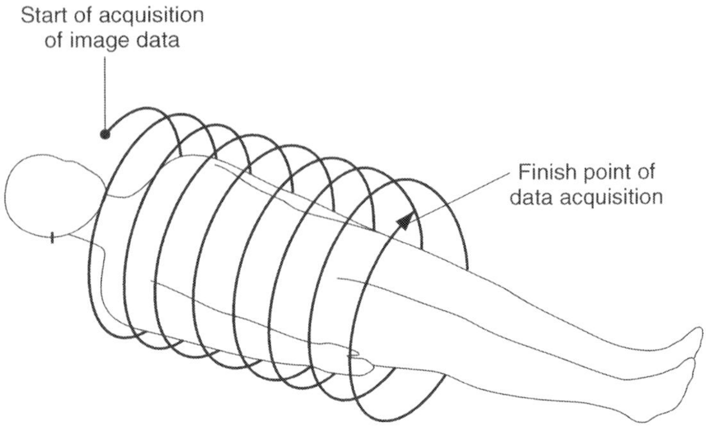

FIGURE 8.3. Diagram of the spiral of data obtained with modern CT scanners.

As the number of detector rows has increased, the volume of the anatomy being imaged with each exposure has also increased. As the multiple slices are all acquired at the same time and are contiguous with the adjacent slice this means that the scanner is effectively obtaining a "volume" of data that corresponds to the same volume of tissue scanned (Fig. 8.3).

Technology has advanced to the point where modern CT scanners are now able to use a large number of detector rows to enable sufficient coverage to image whole anatomical areas in sub-second exposure times. This means that organs such as the heart are now readily accessible to CT imaging as the coverage of the detector rows is such that the whole organ can be included in a single scan and the speed of the image acquisition means that motion artifacts from the heart beating are virtually eliminated.

The very small detectors and thin slices obtained with modern multislice CT scanners result in the use of very small voxels which are isotropic, i.e., they are the same size in all three dimensions. This means that there is no loss in image resolution when viewing the data in any plane. Images can be viewed axially, sagittally, coronally, or in an oblique plane with no loss of resolution (Fig. 8.4). When combined with the fact

a

b

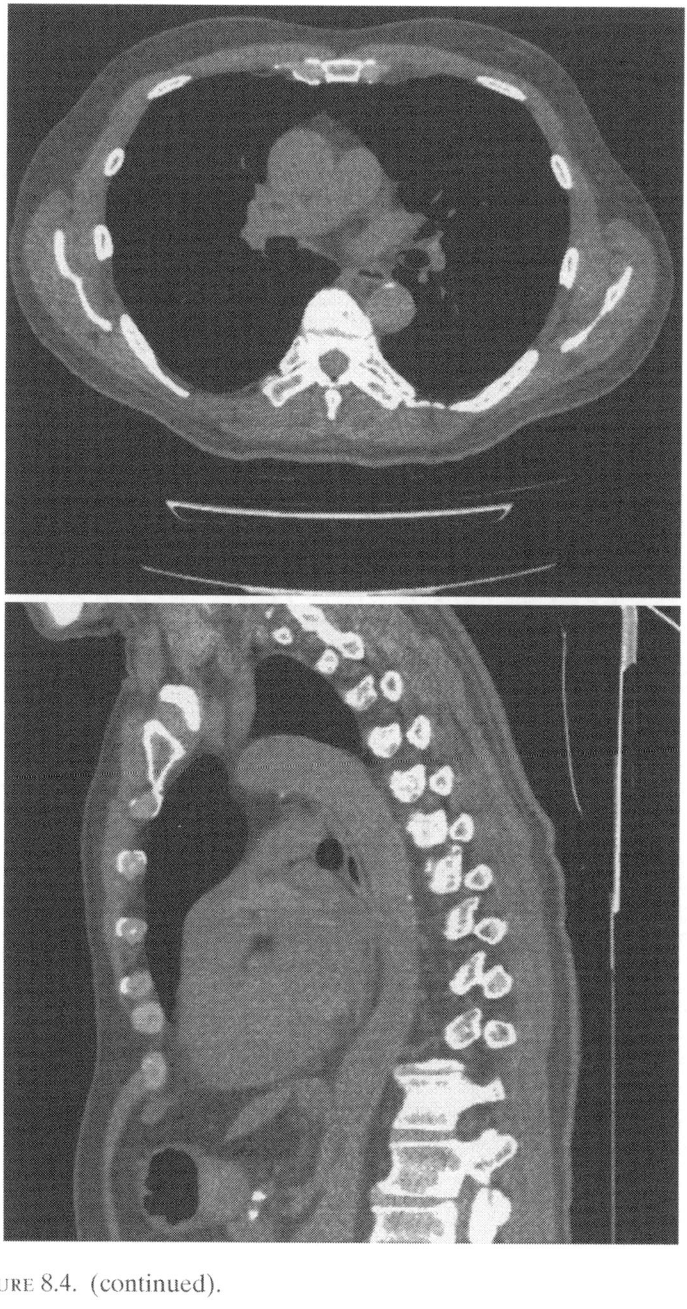

FIGURE 8.4. (continued).

c

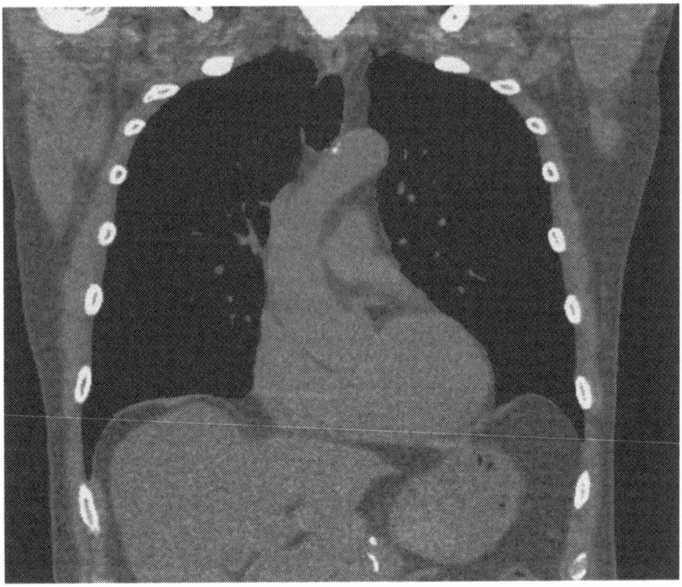

FIGURE 8.4. Examples of the high-quality axial (a), sagittal (b), and coronal (c) images that can be obtained with modern MSCT scanners.

that a volume of data is acquired by the scanner, this makes a modern MSCT scanner a truly multiplanar imaging modality.

The large numbers of thin slices that are generated by modern CT scanners also mean that, in effect, a volume of data has been acquired. These data can then be "volume rendered" to generate 3D images of user-defined anatomy (Fig. 8.5). This is particularly effective in orthopedic imaging but does have its uses for other clinical areas as well.

Once the patient has been scanned and the image data have been acquired, it is possible to apply differing reconstruction techniques which result in images that give differing types of information, e.g., high-resolution algorithms can be applied to the "raw" scan data to provide images with very high spatial resolution. These can be particularly useful in imaging of the lung fields and bony anatomy but results in poor resolution

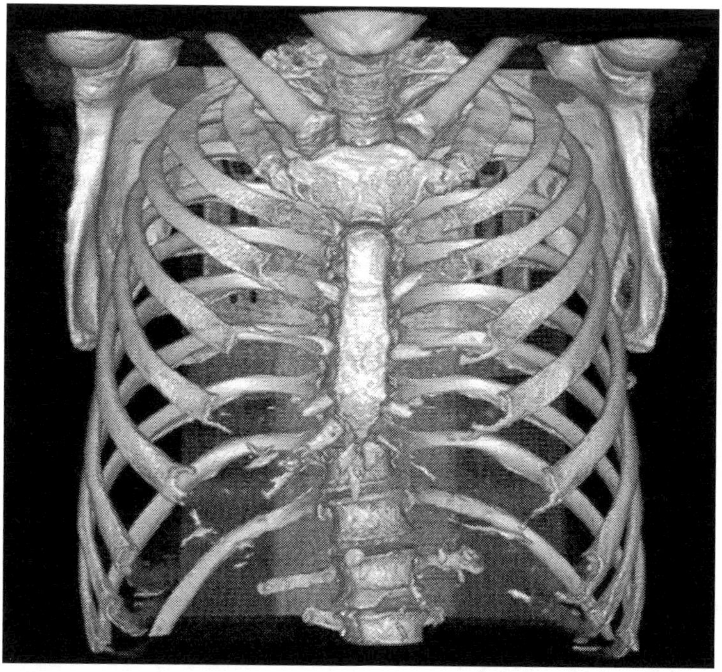

FIGURE 8.5. Example of a volume-rendered image of the bony thorax.

of the soft tissues. Separate soft tissue algorithms are applied to the raw data to obtain images which give a differing set of images that have good soft tissue resolution to enable other organs to be assessed in sufficient detail (Figs. 8.6 and 8.7).

After the image has been reconstructed it can be viewed on a monitor where it can be windowed for viewing. The term "windowing" refers to altering the image viewing settings which enables pixels with the chosen HU values to be seen on the image. Choosing an image window that only includes pixels with a HU value in the lung parenchymal range means that only lung tissue will be visible on the image. If other soft tissues are required to be viewed the selected window can be set

a

b

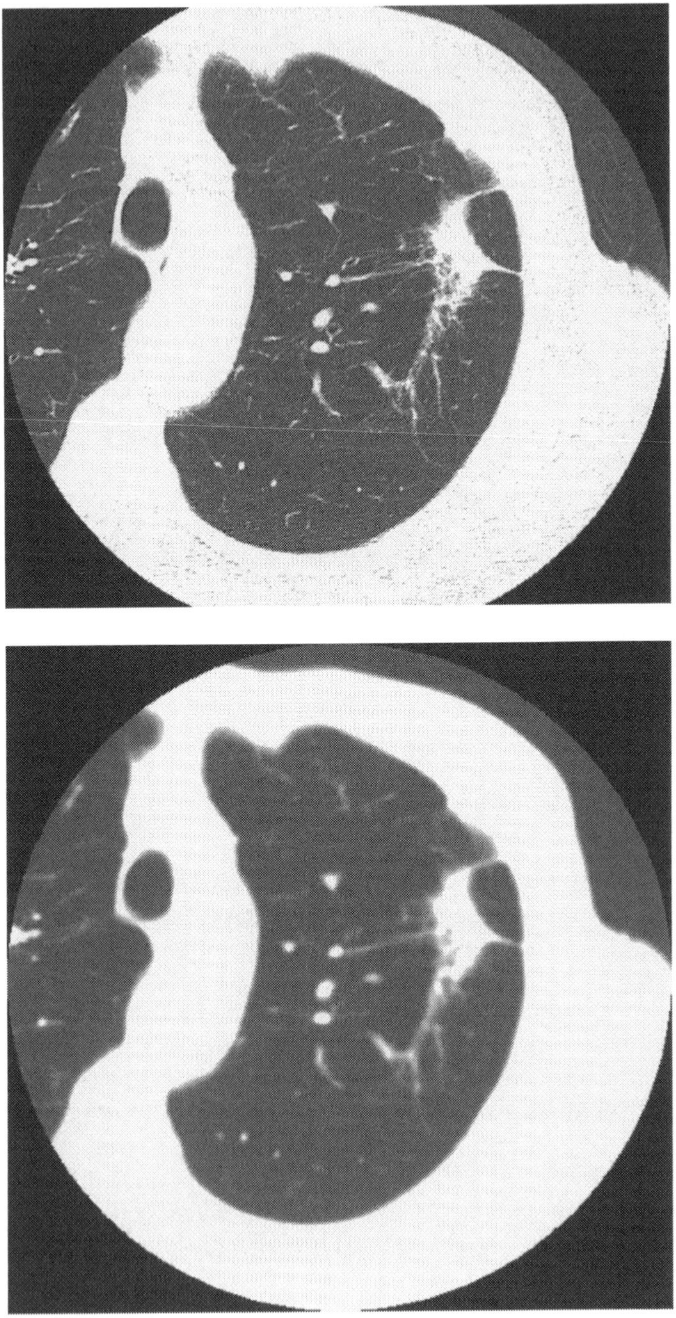

FIGURE 8.6. Examples of the same image of lung parenchyma with high-resolution (a) and soft tissue (b) algorithms applied. This demonstrates the extra information that can be gained within the lung tissue from the use of a higher resolution technique.

to include these. A window can be set to include a very wide range of HU values but this will have very little image contrast as a large number of differing values are spread across the available image gray scale (Fig. 8.8).

a

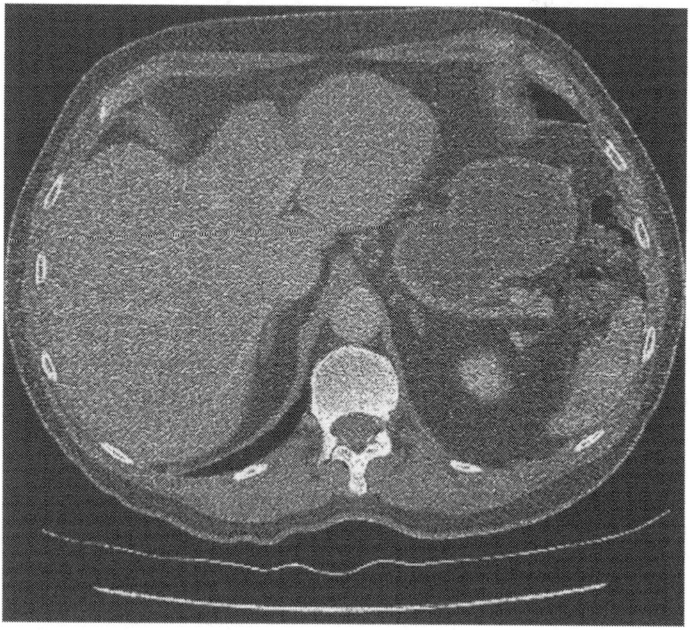

FIGURE 8.7. (continued).

b

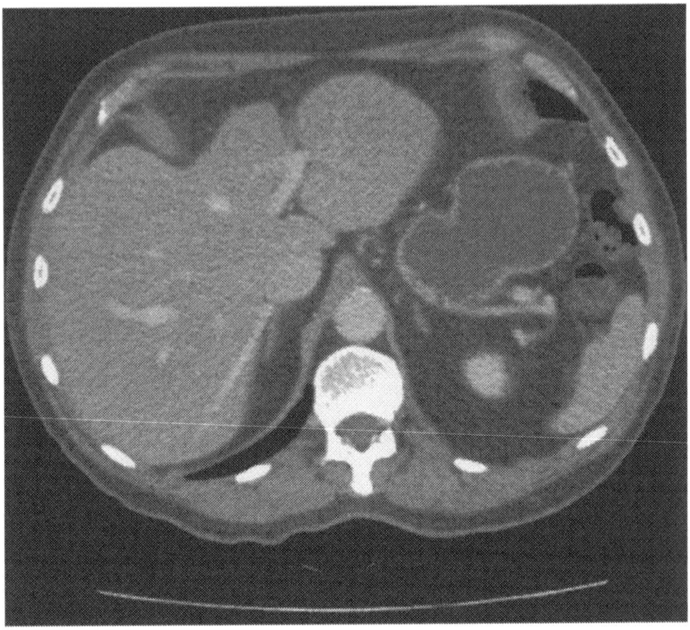

FIGURE 8.7. Examples of the same image of soft tissue organs with high-resolution (a) and soft tissue (b) algorithms applied. This demonstrates the increase in image noise and corresponding loss of tissue detail with the use of a higher resolution technique.

One side effect of the increasing number of detector rows in modern CT scanners is the large increase in the amount of images that are produced for each and every patient. Although modern day Picture Archiving and Communication Systems (PACS) are generally set up with such systems in mind, the increase in the amount of patients being imaged and the increasing amount of images that each examination now produces are having (and will have) a greater and greater impact on these systems.

a

b

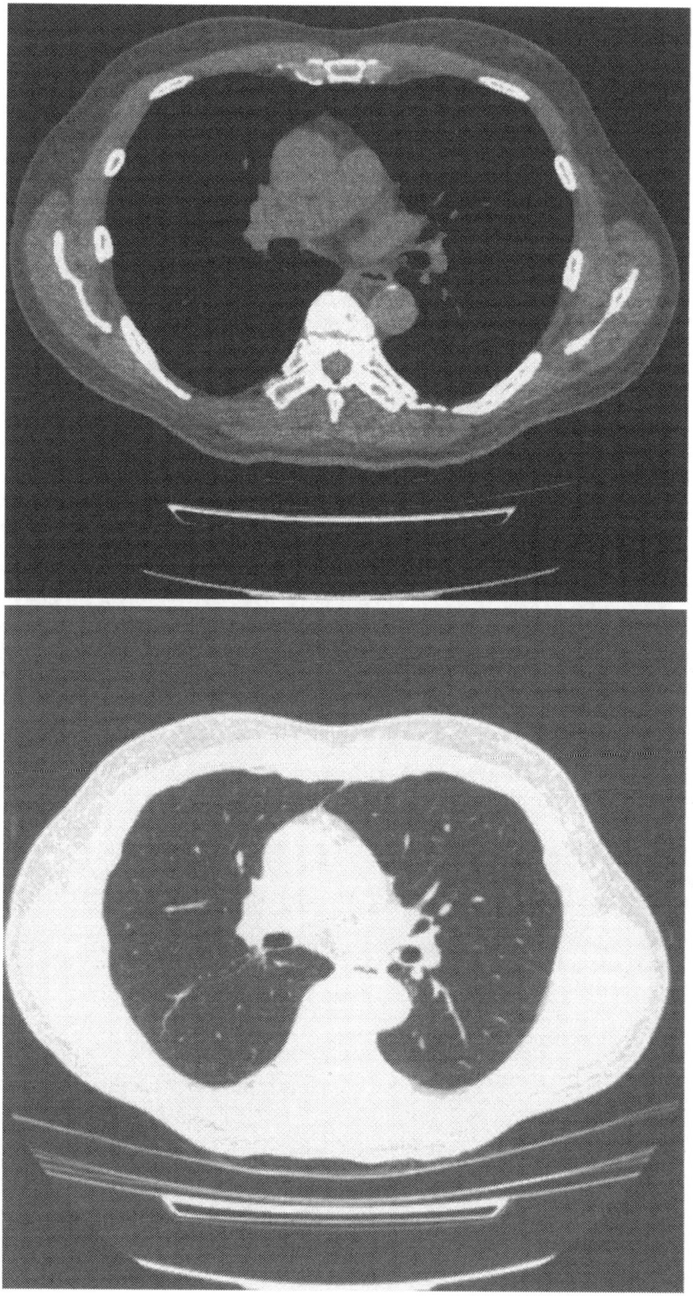

FIGURE 8.8. (continued).

c

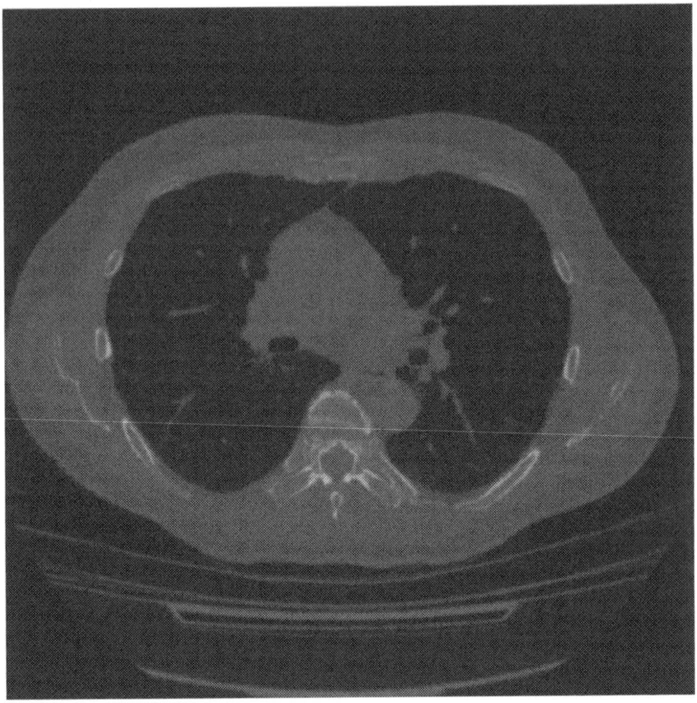

FIGURE 8.8. Examples of the same image windowed with soft tissue (a), lung (b), and very wide (c) windows demonstrating the differing information that can be included or excluded from the image by windowing.

8.1 Intravenous Contrast Agent

Iodinated IV contrast agent is generally used when imaging the soft tissue structures of the thorax and mediastinum as it helps differentiate the vasculature from other soft tissue structures and pathologies, e.g., a blood vessel shown in cross section may have a very similar appearance to an enlarged lymph node. By using IV contrast agent the vessel will enhance to a much greater extent than the node due to the increase in density of the blood because of the contrast agent dispersing within it (Fig. 8.9).

Iodinated IV contrast agent is generally introduced through peripheral IV cannulation with the antecubital vein being the traditionally favored site of venepuncture. The timing of the image acquisition in relation to the injection of the contrast agent is also an important parameter. Should arterial vascular enhancement be required, e.g., for differentiation of an aortic dissection, then the imaging will have to be undertaken quite quickly after the initiation of the injection to ensure a good bolus of contrast agent is present within the vessel of interest. Within the chest this delay tends to be 15–20 s for pulmonary artery enhancement and 20–30 s for thoracic aortic enhancement. These times are, however, dependent upon the cardiac output of the subject. If systemic venous enhancement is required then the start of the scan is delayed by the amount of time that allows the agent to circulate through the capillary bed and back into the venous system. This will generally be in the 60–80 s range (Fig. 8.10).

Modern CT scanners tend to have special software that allows low radiation dose monitoring scans to be undertaken that enable the operators to "see" the contrast agent arriving at a designated point and, therefore, trigger the scan at exactly the optimum moment.

Certain organs and pathologies also take up the agent in differing ways and this is a valuable aid to the diagnosis and interpretation of images. As the contrast agent is further dispersed throughout the blood volume, it loses its bolus effect and gives much less enhancement of the vasculature. This is

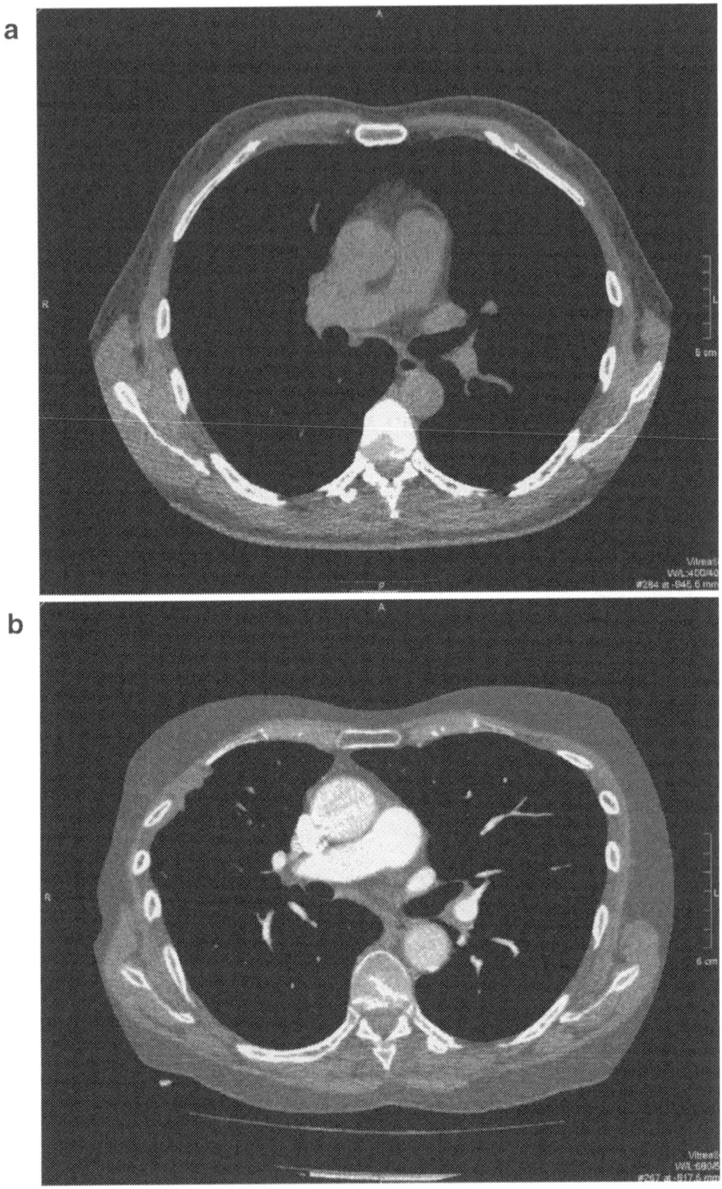

FIGURE 8.9. Examples of an image through the mediastinum without (a) and with (b) IV contrast enhancement.

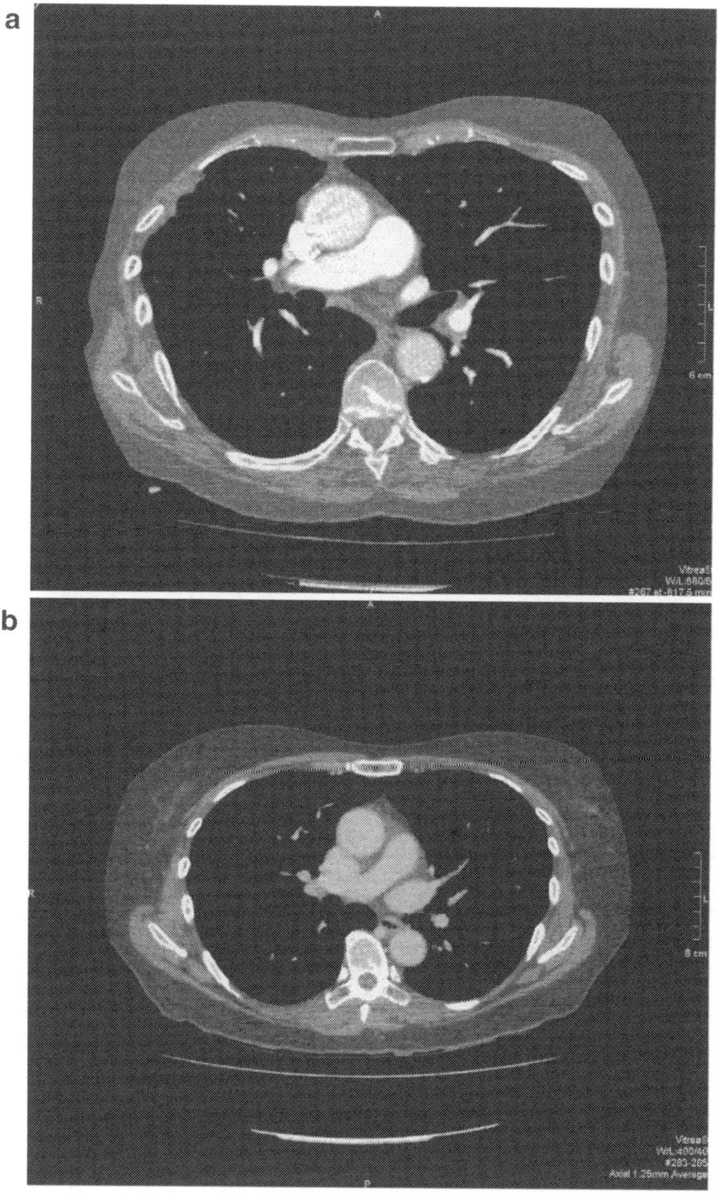

FIGURE 8.10. Examples of an image through the mediastinum with arterial (a) and venous (b) IV contrast enhancement.

further weakened by the kidneys filtering the agent from the blood and passing it into the urinary system to be excreted with the urine. After a few minutes the diagnostic effects of the contrast agent are lost from the majority of the body's vasculature and organs.

CT scanning of the lungs alone does not generally require the use of iodinated IV contrast agent as there is sufficient natural contrast between the air and the lung parenchyma to give sufficient detail. IV contrast agent would add very little extra information for the increased risk associated with its administration.

Although iodinated contrast agent contains iodine within its chemical structure, patient allergy to iodine preparations is rarely a contraindication to its administration, a quoted iodine allergy often being the result of a reaction to skin iodine preparations. It is very unlikely that these patients will have an allergic reaction to IV contrast agent and only a previous history of sensitivity to iodinated IV contrast agent should be considered a contraindication to its future administration.

The administration of IV contrast agent is, however, a potential problem in the renally impaired patient as it may precipitate renal failure in patients with a low glomerular filtration rate leading to contrast-induced nephropathy (CIN).

8.2 Patient Preparation and Positioning

Patients are generally changed into hospital gowns for CT of the thorax to prevent radio opaque objects from degrading the scans, e.g., bra fastenings. Oral contrast agents may be given depending upon which thoracic structures and/or other organs are the main focus of interest, e.g., CT scans for lung fields alone generally do not require any contrast agents present within the oesophagus or stomach as these structures are not the principle area of interest. However, imaging of patients with oesophageal pathology or other pathology that may directly involve or spread to areas surrounding any of the gastrointestinal tract would benefit from having these structures filled with an easily recognizable fluid. Oral contrast agents are usually given in the form of a drink immediately prior to the scan and can either be positive or negative in nature; positive contrast agents appear brighter than the surrounding soft tissues on the images while negative agents appear darker.

The patient is usually positioned supine on the scanner couch so that they pass through the scanner aperture either head or feet first depending on local preferences and traditions. Arms are usually raised onto a pillow or support above the head to prevent the X-ray beam being attenuated by the structure of the upper limb which would result in degradation of the scans of the thorax by streak artifacts across the images. Scanning is usually undertaken during arrested inspiration but imaging of certain lung pathologies may also benefit from comparative scans being taken in arrested expiration to check for air trapping, etc. Scanning in the prone position may also be undertaken to ascertain the effect of gravity on certain structures and/or pathologies. Modern MSCT scanners have no problem with obtaining imaging of the whole of the thorax in a single breath hold which is often of only 2 or 3 s duration. Single breath hold imaging removes the problems of differential inspiratory effort during consecutive scans which may result in areas of tissue not being imaged correctly.

8.3 Radiation Dose

CT is a high radiation dose examination. Although every effort should be undertaken by the radiographers to reduce the dose used during CT scanning, it still gives rise to a much higher absorbed radiation dose than conventional radiography. A typical effective dose for a CT of the chest is approximately 8 millisieverts (mSv) which is equivalent to 3.6 years natural background radiation or 400 chest X-rays; for comparison purposes a normal chest X-ray is 0.02 mSv/3 days background radiation equivalent (UK average = 2.2 mSv per annum with regional variations from 1.5 to 7.5 mSv per annum) [1]. Obviously, the best way to reduce a patient's dose is to not do the scan in the first place so CT scanning should only be undertaken when there are genuine clinical reasons to do so and the result will impact on the patient's management. The scan should also be limited to include only those regions that are clinically under suspicion; including other areas will substantially increase a patients radiation dose, e.g., a CT scan of the chest should not be continued into the abdomen unless there is sufficient suspicion of intra abdominal pathology to warrant it.

8.4 Key Points

1) CT is a high-radiation examination and, therefore, should only be undertaken when the results will affect patient management.
2) Modern MSCT scanners often produce large numbers of images (often many hundreds per patient).
3) Modern MSCT scanners give a volume of data that can be viewed in multiple planes, including 3D rendered images.
4) Iodinated IV contrast agents are often required for CT scans of the thorax.
5) High-resolution images can be obtained for greater lung parenchymal detail.

Reference

1. UK Health Protection Agency (2008) Understanding Radiation: Patient Dose Information, http://hpa.org.uk

Chapter 9
Computed Tomography (CT): Clinical Indications

CT is often the next imaging investigation for abnormalities discovered on a chest X-ray. In this chapter we will give some simple examples of CT abnormality and how a CT may be useful in the further investigation of chest X-ray abnormalities.

CT is very useful for evaluation of abnormalities such as a nodule particularly with the ability of multislice CT scan to give volumetric analysis. This enables the follow-up of a nodule's size over a period of time. Accompanying abnormalities such as mediastinal or hilar lymph node enlargement, which may not be apparent on a chest X-ray, will be seen on a CT scan (Fig. 9.1).

A CT scan of the thorax is generally performed with intravenous contrast and usually includes the upper abdomen, allowing evaluation of the liver, adrenal glands, and para-aortic regions, looking for metastatic disease as this is important in the accurate staging of lung tumours.

CT is also an excellent modality for evaluation of the thoracic aorta in conditions such as dissection or aneurysmal dilatation (Fig. 9.2).

Modern multislice CT scanners are also excellent for evaluation of the pulmonary arteries, particularly in terms of thromboembolic diseases. This is particularly used in patients with an abnormal chest X-ray as nuclear medicine perfusion imaging is less accurate in this case (Fig. 9.3).

Intrinsic abnormalities of the lungs such as interstitial lung disease are well demonstrated by CT, particularly

R. Joarder, N. Crundwell (eds.), *Chest X-Ray in Clinical Practice*,

DOI 10.1007/978-1-84882-099-9_9,

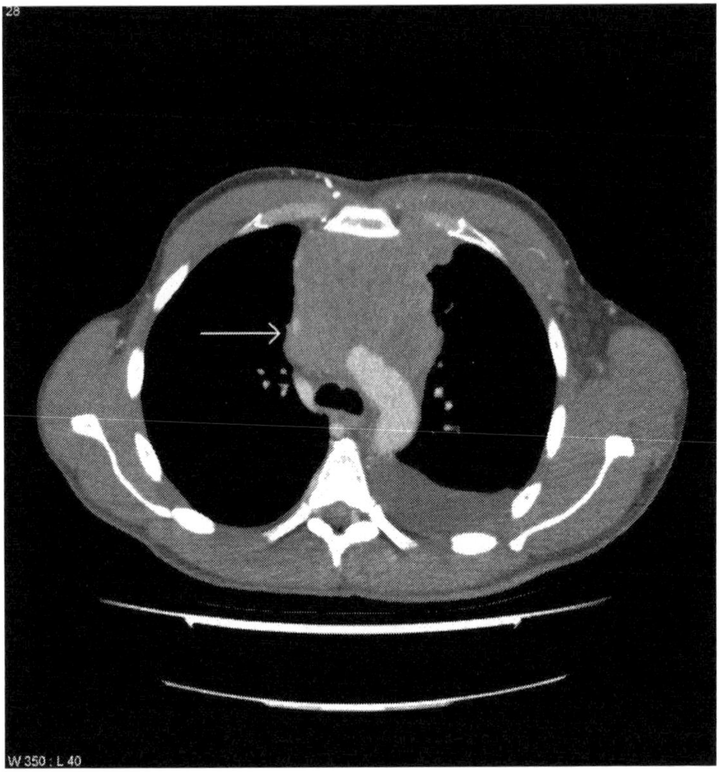

FIGURE 9.1. Lymphoma with extensive mediastinal involvement causing superior vena cava obstruction (arrow).

high-resolution CT. This is performed with a slightly higher dose and a different reconstruction which results in a better definition of structures. Interpretation is complex and beyond the scope of this book. It is, however, commonly used to evaluate the lung parenchyma in such conditions as pulmonary fibrosis, bronchiectasis, sarcoidosis, organizing pneumonias, asbestos-related lung disease, and lymphangitis carcinomatosis (Fig. 9.4).

CT scanning is invaluable in complex trauma, particularly with modern multislice technology when the entire cervical and thoracic spine as well as the thorax can be imaged in seconds.

a

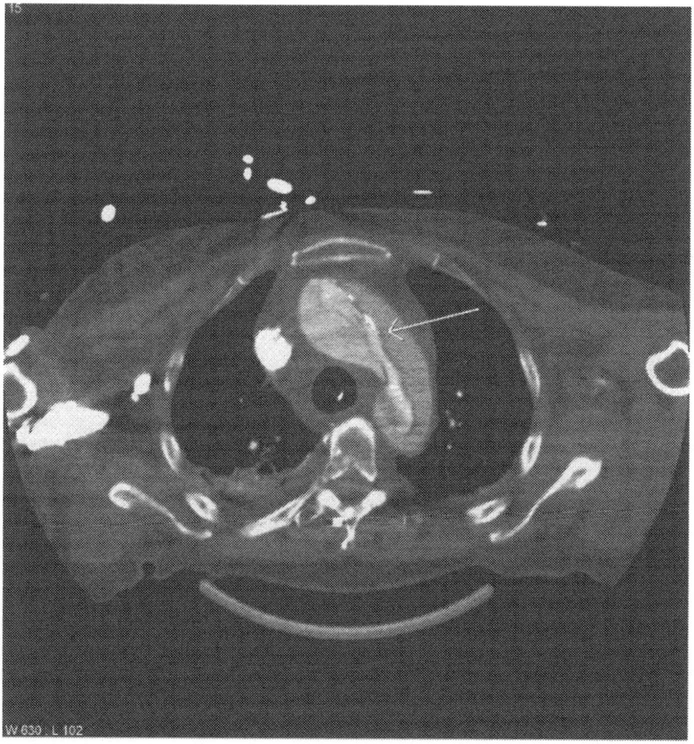

FIGURE 9.2a. Thoracic aortic dissection involving the arch of the aorta. The *arrow* indicates the dissection flap and there is contrast within the true lumen (medial) and none in the false lumen (lateral).

b

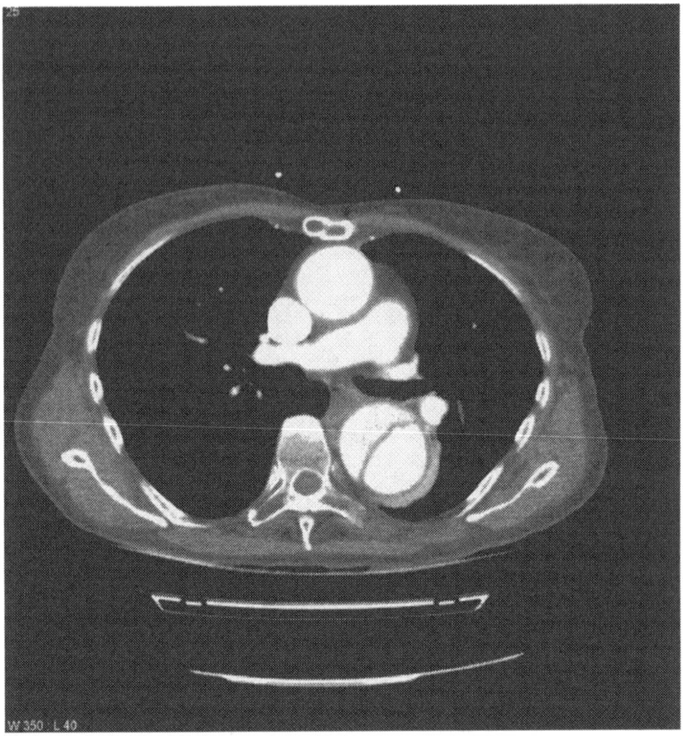

FIGURE 9.2b. Dissection of the descending aorta with the dissection flap giving the descending aorta an appearance similar to a tennis ball. Contrast is present within the true and false lumens.

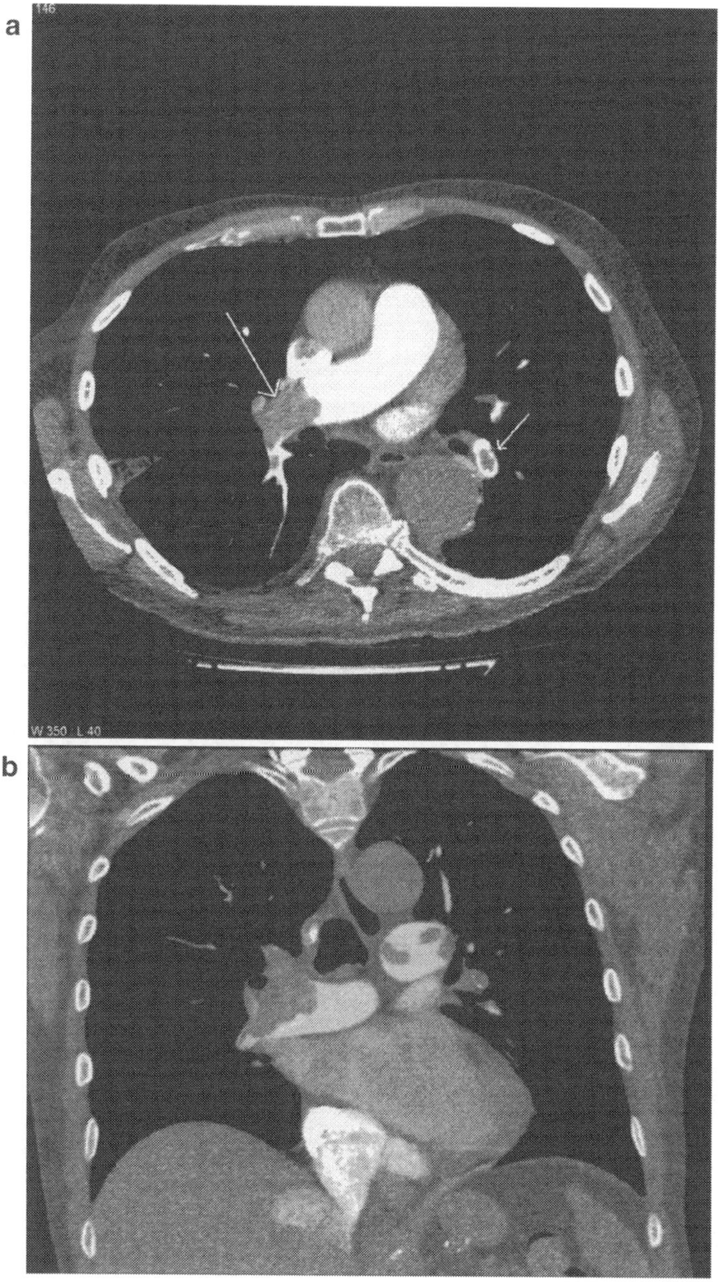

FIGURE 9.3. (a) Axial image of large pulmonary emboli within both main pulmonary arteries (*arrows*); (b) coronal reconstruction.

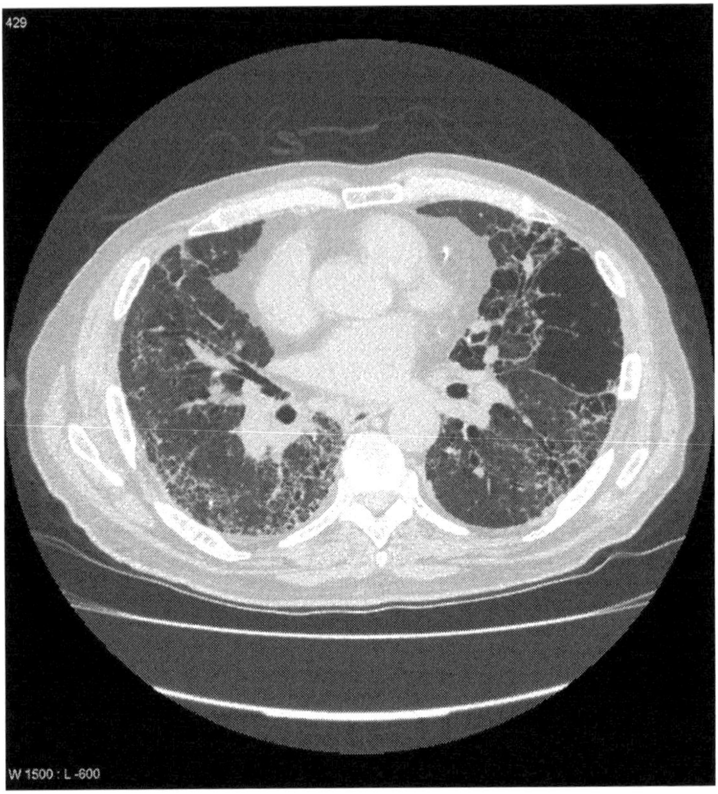

FIGURE 9.4. Pulmonary fibrosis involving the lung bases with peripheral interlobular septal thickening and honeycomb lung.

Index

FSC
www.fsc.org
MIX
Papier | Fördert gute Waldnutzung
FSC® C083411

Kolibri 360 GmbH
Ferdinand-Jühlke-Straße 7
99095 Erfurt, Deutschland
produktsicherheit@kolibri360.de